# INFECTED KIN

## Medical Anthropology: Health, Inequality, and Social Justice

Series editor: Lenore Manderson

Books in the Medical Anthropology series are concerned with social patterns of and social responses to ill health, disease, and suffering, and how social exclusion and social justice shape health and healing outcomes. The series is designed to reflect the diversity of contemporary medical anthropological research and writing, and will offer scholars a forum to publish work that showcases the theoretical sophistication, methodological soundness, and ethnographic richness of the field.

Books in the series may include studies on the organization and movement of peoples, technologies, and treatments, how inequalities pattern access to these, and how individuals, communities and states respond to various assaults on well-being, including from illness, disaster, and violence.

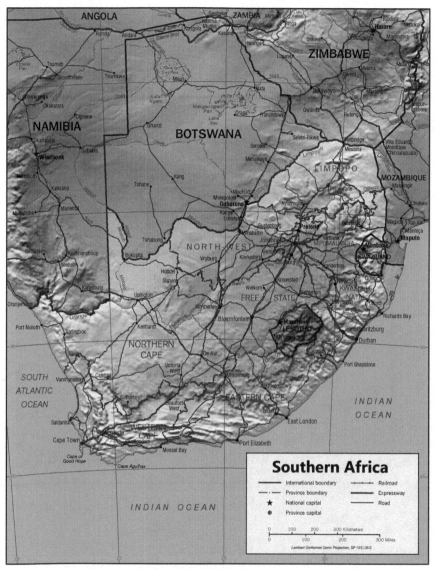

FRONTISPIECE. Map of Southern Africa, noting the location of Lesotho. Courtesy of *The World Factbook* of the Central Intelligence Agency of the United States of America, 2007.

# INFECTED KIN

## Orphan Care and AIDS in Lesotho

ELLEN BLOCK AND WILL MCGRATH

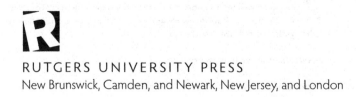

RUTGERS UNIVERSITY PRESS
New Brunswick, Camden, and Newark, New Jersey, and London

Library of Congress Cataloging-in-Publication Data

Names: Block, Ellen (Mary Ellen), author. | McGrath, Will, 1980–author.
Title: Infected kin : orphan care and AIDS in Lesotho / Ellen Block and Will
McGrath.
Description: New Brunswick : Rutgers University Press, 2019. | Series: Medical
Anthropology: Health, Inequality, and Social Justice | Includes bibliographical
references and index.
Identifiers: LCCN 2018035885 | ISBN 9781978804746 (pbk.) | ISBN 9781978804753
(cloth)
Subjects: LCSH: AIDS (Disease)—Lesotho. | AIDS (Disease) in children—
Lesotho. | Orphans—Care—Lesotho. | Families—Lesotho. | Kinship—Lesotho. |
Medical Anthropology.
Classification: LCC RA643.86.L5 B56 2019 | DDC 362.19697/920096885—dc23
LC record available at https://lccn.loc.gov/2018035885

A British Cataloging-in-Publication record for this book is available from the British
Library.

All photos by Ellen Block unless otherwise noted.

∞ The paper used in this publication meets the requirements of the American
National Standard for Information Sciences—Permanence of Paper for Printed
Library Materials, ANSI Z39.48-1992.

www.rutgersuniversitypress.org

Manufactured in the United States of America

For Sam, Eve, and Mara

# CONTENTS

# ILLUSTRATIONS

# FOREWORD

LENORE MANDERSON

Medical Anthropology: Health, Inequality, and Social Justice is a new series from Rutgers University Press designed to capture the diversity of contemporary medical anthropological research and writing. The beauty of ethnography is its capacity, through storytelling, to make sense of suffering as a social experience and to set it in context. Central to our focus in this series on health, illness, inequality, and social justice, therefore, is the way in which social structures and ideologies shape the likelihood and impact of infections, injuries, bodily ruptures and disease, chronic conditions and disability, treatment and care, and social repair and death.

The brief for this series is broad. The books are concerned with health and illness, healing practices, and access to care, but the authors illustrate too the importance of context—of geography, physical condition, service availability, and income. Health and illness are social facts; the circumstances of the maintenance and loss of health are always and everywhere shaped by structural, global, and local relations. Society, culture, economy, and political organization, as much as ecology, shape the variance of illness, disability, and disadvantage. But as medical anthropologists have long illustrated, the relationships between social context and health status are complex. In addressing these questions, the authors in this series showcase the theoretical sophistication, methodological rigor, and empirical richness of the field while expanding a map of illness and social and institutional life to illustrate the effects of material conditions and social meanings in troubling and surprising ways.

The books in the series move across social circumstances, health conditions, and geography, as well as their intersections and interactions, to demonstrate how individuals, communities, and states manage assaults on well-being. The books reflect medical anthropology as a constantly changing field of scholarship, drawing diversely on research in residential and virtual communities, clinics, and laboratories; in emergency care and public health settings; with service providers, individual healers, and households; and with social bodies, human bodies, and biologies. While medical anthropology once concentrated on systems of healing, particular diseases, and embodied experiences, today, the field has expanded to include environmental disaster and war, science, technology and faith, gender-based violence, and forced migration. Curiosity about the body and its vicissitudes remains a pivot for our work, but our concerns are with the location of bodies in social life and with how social structures, temporal imperatives, and shifting exigencies shape life courses. This dynamic field reflects an ethics of the discipline to address these pressing issues of our time.

Globalization has contributed to and adds to the complexity of influences on health outcomes; it (re)produces social and economic relations that institutionalize poverty, unequal conditions of everyday life and work, and environments in which diseases increase or subside. Globalization patterns the movement and relations of peoples, technologies and knowledge, and programs and treatments; it shapes differences in health experiences and outcomes across space; and it informs and amplifies inequalities at individual and country levels. Global forces and local inequalities compound and constantly load on individuals to impact their physical and mental health and their households and communities. At the same time, as the subtitle of this series indicates, we are concerned with questions of social exclusion and inclusion and social justice and repair—again, both globally and in local settings. The books will challenge readers to reflect not only on sickness and suffering, deficit and despair but also on resistance and restitution—on how people respond to injustices and evade the fault lines that might seem to predetermine life outcomes. While not all of the books take this direction, the aim is to widen the frame within which we conceptualize embodiment and suffering.

For some 35 years now, HIV and AIDS have dominated medical anthropology and shaped the theories and methods we use and the trajectories of our careers in health and illness. The virus and its modes of infection, its prevention and management, its risk factors and vulnerabilities, and its socialities and fallouts have shaped the narratives of changing epidemiologies, demographies, and economies. The virus has exposed the fault lines between as well as within nations, illustrating not only how infection tracks the movement and relations of people but also the susceptibility of people to structures and institutions at multiple levels: the globalization of policies to control HIV's spread, the travel of ideas that have shaped public and sexual health programs, the power of corporate interests to manipulate the availability and accessibility of lifesaving medication, and the energies of social movements to battle the impact of infection. But at the same time, HIV is felt very locally and intimately, shaping people's personal lives, their own health, and the health of those closest to them: children, lovers and spouses, siblings, parents, and grandparents. HIV is, Ellen Block and Will McGrath show us, a kinship disease.

In *Infected Kin: Orphan Care and AIDS in Lesotho*, Block and McGrath take us to the rural highlands of Lesotho in southern Africa. Lesotho is a small and impoverished country, landlocked by and economically dependent on South

Africa via the provision of water to industrial South Africa and remittances from migrant workers. Workers were recruited first from Lesotho's own rural communities to South Africa's mines (gold and diamond); more recently, people have sought employment in South Africa's large service economy. HIV's introduction to Lesotho more than three decades ago occurred in association with this population flow. Nearly 25 percent of its adult population is now infected with HIV, with reverberations throughout communities as people of reproductive and productive ages have died from complications of infection. Many of their children too have died—evidence of how the virus continues to exploit the vulnerabilities of poor living conditions, food insecurity, and poor access to medical care. But first, with the death of their parents, these children—and other children not infected—are cared for, as well as possible, within the circles of their kin.

*Infected Kin* takes us into the households and intimate lives of children orphaned by AIDS to illustrate the power of the family and the primacy of kin-based care to ward off the desolations of orphanhood and disease. Each chapter begins with a literary nonfiction vignette written by Will McGrath: powerful, often magical accounts that breathe life into the settlements of Lesotho and the men, women, and children who live there. We readers are captured by the affects of place, relationship, temperament, and circumstance; as we are so engaged, Ellen Block then takes over, providing us with a sharp ethnographic account of how everyday understandings of relatedness and obligation shape people's lives, well-being, and personal care. The result is uniquely engaging. We mourn Matseli's death, and we have barely got to know him; we sympathize deeply with grandmothers 'M'e Masekha and 'M'e Masello as they care for children and struggle to keep their families together despite their erosion by AIDS. "Family," Will McGrath writes, "is just an idea." Ellen Block shows us how this is so and how this idea is honored under the most trying conditions.

# PREFACE
## On Collaboration and Suffering

I—Ellen—have been thinking about how to represent suffering for a long time. It emerged shortly after returning from my first two months of fieldwork in 2007, when friends would ask me about my trip to Lesotho. I would give the elevator-pitch version—I was doing research on the impact of AIDS on orphans and their caregivers—and they frequently reacted with some variation of "That must be so sad." And while some extremely difficult things happened to people I care about, and while their suffering is real and needs to be recounted and addressed, the days were also filled with hilarity, raunchiness, boredom, and the pleasantly mundane rhythms of life in rural Lesotho. My husband and collaborator, Will McGrath, a literary nonfiction writer, has chronicled the verbal jousting and elaborate genial shenanigans that his colleagues at the local high school in Mokhotlong engaged him in daily—the same teachers whose lives have been ravaged by HIV; who chopped wood after school for fellow teachers' funeral feasts; whose sons, daughters, and spouses migrated to South Africa for work and returned with more than remittances.

How do I write a book about AIDS and orphans without falling prey to what Nigerian author Chimamanda Ngozi Adichie calls "the danger of the single story" (2009)? In a more earnest and less sarcastic version of Binyavanga Wainaina's "How to Write about Africa" (2006), Adichie argues that the "single story" of Africans, which emphasizes suffering, leaves "no possibility of feelings more complex than pity, no possibility of a connection as human equals." As Joel Robbins (2013) recently noted, the turn to the "suffering slot" in anthropology was in many ways inevitable. People's suffering and our own complicity in it were brought to light—or at the very least, finally acknowledged—and could no longer be ignored. Anthropology could no longer in good conscience focus on theoretical questions of comparatively little import. At the same time, Robbins has highlighted the necessity of moving away from exclusively focusing on suffering by emphasizing what he calls "an anthropology of the good" (Robbins 2013). He thinks anthropologists should illuminate the ways in which "people living in different societies strive to create good in their lives" (Robbins 2013, 457).

What follows here is surely an inadequate attempt to combat Adichie's single story while at the same time conveying the real and important tales of loss and suffering that abound in rural Lesotho, where a quarter of adults are infected with HIV. One way I hope to counteract the danger of the single story and to make my work eminently readable for scholars, students, and the wider public is by incorporating literary elements into this book. Threading the literary into the ethnographic is, in many ways, a direct response to Adichie's and Robbins' calls to action. I take Adichie's prohibition of the single story literally: each chapter of this book begins with a vignette written by my husband, Will McGrath. In addition to being my spouse, Will has the benefit of being a nonfiction writer. He accompanied me for almost all of my time in Lesotho, at times teaching at the local high school, at times writing, and at times caring for our young children.

Will and I believe that adding clearly delineated elements of literary nonfiction to rigorous scholarship can enhance a reader's understanding of the experiences of those living with HIV in Lesotho. Literary nonfiction draws much of its power from its ability to be evocative—silences, omissions, and a lack of *saying* are very important modes of communication. Done properly, the blank space between sections or a question left unanswered can have more power than a page of descriptive text. Academic writing by its nature does not have the luxury of *not saying*. The whole point is to *say*. But literary writing can make powerful use of evocation in its etymological sense—calling forth or summoning—using prose that draws out other meanings and connotations. This evocativeness expects the reader's interpretation, roots the response personally in the reader in a manner that moves away from passive listening, and aims for an active construction of meaning in the text—drawing the reader into deeper empathetic connection with the people of Mokhotlong, who are at the heart of this scholarship.

Literary nonfiction also takes liberties with the notion of "time." Some of the vignettes that open these chapters deliberately fracture a standard linear chronology. This kind of authorial withholding can ultimately lead to deeper insight. The way we readers understand the world very rarely works in a straight line. We construct meaning in recursive loops: we go back over old memories, old information, and glean new insights—working not in a linear fashion but from multiple jagged approaches. We are notoriously good at talking around the point, at coming at something obliquely—an evasiveness that can reveal more about a situation than a straightforward telling might. A literature intent on understanding humans benefits from utilizing these same very human techniques.

Literary nonfiction has the built-in assumption that a full human portraiture benefits from a multilayered mode of writing. From the smallest scale of word choice and punctuation to symbols and allusions and to the largest scale of structure, theme, and mood—literary writing relies on layering elements to produce a fully realized portrait of a person, who by nature is defined by many layers: physical, mental, emotional, moral, psychological, cultural, and more.

Human beings are so complex that we need all our creative resources to catch just a glimpse—to avoid Adichie's "single story."

By fusing literary nonfiction and scholarship—using two distinct voices, modes, and perspectives—we hope to move beyond the "single story." In the nonfiction vignettes, we draw on the elements of literary writing that allow for the coevalness of joy and pain, spotlighting moments of ethnographic import and celebrating the mundane human details of everyday life. When scholars focus too closely on human suffering, the holism and humanism of classic anthropology is often lost. In drawing on the toolkit of creative writers, we can expand on the holistic nature of the discipline and use multiple disciplinary strategies to get closer to the human experience. In this way, while we may not have achieved an "anthropology of the good," as Robbins suggests, we are attempting to achieve an anthropology of the whole.

This book is largely written by the primary author and anthropologist (Ellen). Throughout the book, I employ the first-person singular to indicate me alone. When I use *we*, I am explicit about who that entails—at times I write *we* to refer to Will and me and at times to refer to my research assistant or one of my interlocutors and me. Will is the sole author of the nonfiction vignettes, which appear at the start of each chapter. Likewise, he uses the first-person to refer to himself alone and otherwise clarifies those of whom he writes. The names of all people and some places have been changed for purposes of anonymity.

# ABBREVIATIONS

**AIDS:** acquired immunodeficiency syndrome

**ART:** antiretroviral therapy

**ARV:** antiretroviral

**CD4:** cluster of differentiation 4 (the CD4 count test is used to assess the strength of the immune system of a person living with HIV/AIDS)

**HIV:** human immunodeficiency virus

**MCS:** Mokhotlong Children's Services

**NGOs:** nongovernmental organizations

**PEPFAR:** President's Emergency Plan for AIDS Relief (United States)

**PMTCT:** prevention of mother-to-child transmission

**TB:** tuberculosis

**UNAIDS:** Joint United Nations Programme on HIV/AIDS

**UNICEF:** United Nations Children's Fund (previously named United Nations International Children's Emergency Fund)

**VCT:** voluntary counseling and testing

**WHO:** World Health Organization

# INFECTED KIN

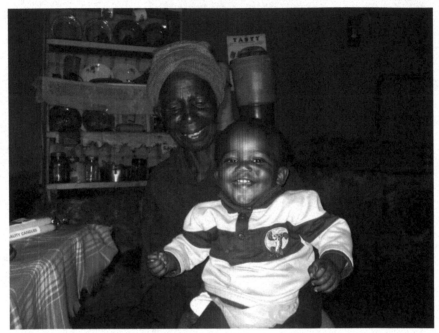

FIGURE I.1. Matseli and his grandmother, 'M'e Maliehi, in their home, Mokhotlong, 2009

# INTRODUCTION
## AIDS Is a Kinship Disease

## *A Story about* Joala[1]

*This is a story about* joala—*or at least I think it is.*

*I should start then by explaining* joala. *I know you don't know what it is because I barely know what it is, and I've had buckets of the stuff.* Joala *is Basotho-style corn beer or corn liquor or corn something. And to be precise, it's actually maize beer, not corn beer, although it is occasionally sorghum beer.*

*Generally speaking, though, you cannot speak generally about* joala. *Each* joala *is its own precious snowflake of intoxicant. I've had* joala *that was the pale color of dead skin, and I've had* joala *that looked like orange juice. I've sipped it from old coffee cans, sipped it from cereal bowls, and sipped it from a jug passed around the village hearth. There is no consistent* joala *experience.*

*The best* joala *I ever had was the brew 'M'e Malereko cooked up in a rinsed-out laundry-detergent bucket. That batch sat behind a couch for two weeks, keeping its own counsel in the dark. When Malereko finally unveiled it at Nthabiseng's birthday party, it had mellowed into a lovely apricot color, sweet and winy on the tongue. At the birthday party, as I watched Nthabiseng and her siblings do a synchronized hop-step routine to pulsing clubby* kwaito *music, I dipped my cup into the communal barrel and watched raisins bob to the surface. They looked like tiny dried mermaids coming up to wave hello. Hello, little mermaids, I said to no one in particular.*

\* \* \*

*Eventually, though, talking about* joala *is always talking about Matseli, he of oversized noggin and joyous drooling grin.*

*Matseli is one of the 40-odd children who, during a typical year, pass through Mokhotlong Children's Services, or MCS. Some children stay here for weeks or months, some longer, until they can be safely reunited with extended family. Most of them are* here because they have lost at least one of their parents. All of them are here because AIDS has rearranged the accepted tenets of how their childhood should work.

Matseli (like so many before him) arrives at the safe home a pre-corpse. He is HIV positive, a hollow-eyed skeleton with an oxygen mask engulfing his face. He lingers around the edges of death just long enough to ruin everyone's month.

And then he recovers.

Gradually, gradually, Matseli's body adjusts to antiretroviral meds. His metabolism stabilizes. He acquires muscle mass and bone density. Later he learns to walk, which is what many children his age would have done a year prior. When I comment on this transformation, Nthabiseng, the managing director of MCS, yells at me, as she will do.

"Hey, uena! Don't you know—this place is where we turn babies into balloons!" She draws out the double-oh sound in the word balloons, inflating those vowels in the same way that she inflates the children.

The better part of a year passes. Now Matseli is a fat and yowling toddler-tank. He is a doe-eyed bruiser, a knocker-down of children, a goofy, stumbling future rugby star. The mental image of his initial form—that skeletal pre-corpse—is crumpled up and pitched into the wastebasket of unpleasant memories.

And finally, after a year, Matseli is healthy enough to return to his maternal grandparents, who live in a small village about an hour's drive from Mokhotlong.

Do I need to tell you that both of his parents are dead?

* * *

We inch our 4WD along the edge of a gorge, tilting far above a valley where small goats caper over scree and other shards of loose terrain. Ellen and I are heading for the rondavel of Ma and Pa Ntho, rheumatic and hilarious maternal grandparents to Matseli and his four siblings. We have come for joala.

See, this is how Ma and Pa Ntho make their living: brewing joala in large stinking barrels in their hut to sell to neighbors—just one of the ways that people can scrape together a living in an earthen hut on the side of a mountain in eastern Lesotho, notoriously devoid of arable land and distinctly cordoned-off from agricultural ease-of-life.

As we approach, they stand in the doorway, looking like a Basotho version of American Gothic. Pa Ntho puts his arm around Ma's shoulders and introduces her—mosali oaka, my wife—indulging in a kind of open affection that is rare between married couples in Lesotho. Years later, Ma Ntho would confide in Ellen—in a conversation about marriage and relationships—that she wished she hadn't gotten hitched so young. She was 15 or 16, doesn't remember which, and is now into her 70s. But then Ma Ntho backtracked. "He is very handsome," she said, smiling, "and we are very caring to each other."

Today, Pa Ntho grins proudly as he presents his wife. She laughs like a teenager and welcomes us inside. On a nearby branch, a white scrap of cloth flutters in the breeze, indicating that home brew is available.

Okay, I should admit that our visit does not revolve entirely around joala. We have come mostly because we miss Matseli, that little piss-and-vinegar destructoid, and somewhat because we need a joala fix but also because we are bearing a stopgap supply of his antiretroviral meds.

Ma and Pa Ntho, in addition to keeping Matseli happy, healthy, coddled, and clean, have also mastered his HIV regimen—a precisely timed and dizzying daily concoction of Medicine X, Suspension Y, and Syrup Z—despite the fact that neither can read and neither have received even the most rudimentary medical education. But today, they have gotten word to Nthabiseng that Matseli's med supply will run out before their next chance to get to the rural clinic, a several-hour hike beyond their village.

Inside the hut, Matseli has just woken from a nap. He is disoriented and—perhaps understandably—begins screaming when he sees us. Ma Ntho slings him onto her back and wraps him in a blanket, assuring him that we have not come to reclaim him for MCS. Soon, in the comfort of Ma Ntho's swaddling, Matseli begins mugging and making faces at us. We swoon. Something about his enormous inverted pyramid of a head, which threatened always to topple him over backward, something about his brute and oblivious pinball trajectory through the other children as he chased a rolling ball, something about his skeleton-to-calzone transformation, like a perverse before-and-after photo—it all inspired the crushing desire to wrap him in your arms and tuck him deeply inside your clothing.

As we hand over the ARVs (antiretroviral drugs),[2] Ma Ntho offers us a seat—a cylindrical chunk of chopped log—and takes a moment to check the rondavel's ancient wind-up clock against Ellen's wristwatch. Matseli's grandmother is punctilious about the timing of his meds, but a hut lacking electricity provides obstacles in this matter.

Now that business is done, it is time to sample the joala. Ma Ntho—with her imperious eyes and mouth perpetually on the horizon of an outright smile—skips over to the giant barrel of joala stewing in the corner. Matseli humors us as we pull him onto our laps. His chunky body has regained that deep country scent, an intoxicating perfume of soil, rain, hay, sweat, minerals, and cook-fire smoke. I nuzzle my face into the tight tiny coils of his hair; he smells like a rutabaga freshly plucked from the earth.

We show Ma Ntho the bucket we have brought with us: a small cornflower-blue pail that a child might take to the beach, able to hold a half gallon of seawater or a half gallon of Basotho moonshine. Joala is always BYO container. Pa Ntho takes the bucket from us, dips it into the murky vat, fills it to the brim, and puts the lid back on. Then he scoops up an extra cup's worth for us to taste.

*We sip the joala carefully, pass it around the room, and smile with delight. "It is excellent," we say.*

*It is not excellent.*

*I have come to realize that the batch 'M'e Malereko cooked up—the sweet, winy raisin brew—was the exception, perhaps wasn't even joala at all. Real village joala is uniformly terrible. Take, for instance, this batch: it is a sour, porridge-like aberration. It has the tang of turned dairy, a cream-of-leek viscosity, and the scent of old carpet. Small mysterious chunks bob in and out of sight. Scraps of maize husk float by on their way to hell. The aftertaste is distinctly that of cured meats—perhaps a fine Genoa salami—salty and fatty and clinging to the tongue.*

*We drink it down and sigh contentedly. We have never tasted something so sublime.*

*Now—too soon, too soon—it is time to go. We collect our joala pail and chat a few extra minutes in our hybrid Engli-Sotho. We take turns hugging Matseli and smothering him with kisses. We head out the door, past the crowd of curious milling neighbors, past the tree branch with the scrap of white cloth, past the gorge and the scrabbling mountain goats, and then home. And only once on the road back does the joala bucket nearly explode, the plastic lid bulging, suddenly domelike—this noncarbonated brew—pulsing and expanding from the unknowable reactions taking place inside.*

* * *

Now we have reached the end of this story about joala.

I suppose I had hoped we wouldn't get here—hoped maybe we'd get sidetracked or wander down the mountain trails of some other story. I thought maybe I could talk around the point for long enough or tell this story like it really was just about joala, even though I knew it really wasn't.

Some time has passed since our visit. Over the Easter holiday—we will learn this later—Matseli begins having diarrhea. He is sick but not terribly so. Ma and Pa Ntho decide they will take him into the rural clinic as soon as it reopens after the holiday weekend.

Ma Ntho sets out on foot early Monday morning, trekking several hours through the mountains with Matseli swaddled to her back. When she arrives, she unwraps the blanket and passes Matseli gently to the nurses. Surely, the nurses can see that he is already dead. Ma Ntho must understand this as well.

Only a few days have passed since he became sick. He never even seemed very ill, she tells us later, just suddenly gone, his quiet little body asleep.

Later that day, Ma and Pa Ntho send word to the extended family of Matseli's dead father, the relatives who—according to Basotho kinship rules—have rights to the child's body, this child they haven't attempted to care for or know in any way.

A day passes before members of the dead father's family arrive to reclaim him. They take him and bury him without a funeral in another village. Pa Ntho travels by *donkey to see the child buried, then returns, upset that they haven't marked the grave or even used a coffin.*

*"Just a wooden box," he says. "If they didn't want to bury him, we would bury him." This is how the other family sends Matseli into the earth.*

\* \* \*

It has been a month now since Matseli's death. Ellen continues to visit Ma and Pa Ntho, even though MCS's business with them has technically concluded. Ellen tells them stories about his time at the safe home, about how much everyone loved him there. When she heads out their way on her motorcycle, Ma and Pa Ntho grow happy; they can hear her coming through the gorge, the motorcycle announcing her presence with its onomatopoetic Sesotho name: se-tu-tu-tu.

Today, Ellen has gone to the Ntho's village to help with the harvest, and they sit sharing a small meal at midday. Ma says she has a little ritual now that makes it easier to start her day. When she wakes up, before first light has crept into the room, she begins to mimic Matseli's tiny voice, calling out for his sister to set the kettle boiling— It is late. It is late. Go out!—just like he used to do each morning. Even in death, he commands them; even in death, he bends them to his indomitable toddler will.

But Pa is still angry, upset at the father's side of the family and their failure to abide by cultural expectations.

"Ache! She wasn't being well cared for," he says, referring to his daughter, Matseli's mother. "She left her husband's home because that family was not caring for her. And when she died, Matseli came to live with us, even though it was the other family's responsibility, having paid likhomo."

Ma chimes in, "Matseli's father—before he died, he was useless! I had to care for my daughter, giving her food and clothing, and he did nothing."

"No one was caring for them there," Pa says again, "and this is why we took in Matseli and his siblings. That other family didn't come to visit; they didn't even know what was happening—even when Matseli was with you at MCS, they didn't know or care."

A silence settles over the group. Over the years, Ma and Pa have watched both of their own children and now one of their grandchildren die.

"God is sometimes doing it like that," Pa says after a moment. "We have one axe to cut all the leaves—but sometimes it can just cut through the small ones and leave the strong ones behind."

\* \* \*

Here's a memory I have of him.

Matseli—his name means "condolences"—is throwing a tantrum, screaming hysterically about something, probably nothing at all. He is wearing a pink and purple shirt that someone has donated, the words Little Princess stamped in rhinestones *across the front. I take him in my arms and leave the MCS nursery; we walk the hallways until he is calm.*

*We walk into Nthabiseng's empty office. I stand up on a chair, still holding him, so we can look out the high windows at the edges of the ceiling.*

*Suddenly, Matseli is entranced, staring out at the land around him, captivated by the pickup trucks on the road, the meandering cattle, the children playing down by the river, and the innumerable darting birds. He looks back at me, eyes wide: Are you seeing this? He stares up at the sky, pupils dilating. Then he looks back into the room, notices the ceiling just inches from his head, and reaches a cautious hand up to touch it. His gaze keeps shifting from the dimensionless blue span of the sky to the firm yellow plaster of the ceiling.*

*He looks at me in wonderment, trying to parse these two concepts—how funny it is, how strange, that there is ceiling above us, just over our heads, where there should be sky.*

-WM-

\* \* \*

## AIDS IS A KINSHIP DISEASE

In many ways, Matseli's story is representative of the challenges faced by AIDS orphans and their caregivers in rural southern Africa. The proximal cause of Matseli's death—dehydration—may have been avoidable, but the structural inequalities that underlie the distal problems faced by Matseli and his family often appear intractable. Structural inequalities are the "steep grades of social inequality" (Farmer 2004, 307) that are rooted in social and economic structures, which place differential value on groups of people. These unequal structures lead to structural violence—violence that is "exerted systematically" by the "social machinery of oppression," causing harm, illness, and sometimes death (Farmer 2004, 307). In Lesotho, widespread poverty, food insecurity, poor job prospects, low educational opportunities, and an entrenched remittance economy make perfect companions for the spread of infectious diseases such as HIV. These challenges have long existed in Lesotho, yet the rapid and devastating emergence of HIV/AIDS has exacerbated all of them. I will return to Matseli and his caregivers later in this chapter, but his experience is emblematic of the multiple and intersecting ways in which AIDS is intertwined with kinship. The threads of his story—along with those of many other families in rural Mokhotlong—will weave throughout this book.

At its most basic level, AIDS's impact on kinship goes beyond the sick individual to pervade the entire social network. While many important studies have highlighted the biomedical realities of HIV as they intersect with cultural, social, and structural factors, I take as my main premise that AIDS is fundamentally a kinship disease. While HIV can be contracted through casual sexual encounters, it spreads through families, sexual lines, and interpersonal relationships in ways that other deadly infectious diseases do not. More important, however, AIDS permeates all facets of social life as it reconfigures and intertwines with kinship. AIDS infects families as much as it infects the body, which is why responses to prevention and treatment efforts are rarely straightforward. An understanding of the knotty relationship between HIV and kinship can explain why people attempt to minimize the social impacts of the disease, even at the cost of their own health. If AIDS had no bearing on relationships, sexual lives, procreative practices, networks of care, and livelihoods, it would be far easier to manage. Yet it does carry these grave implications, particularly in rural Lesotho, where no single family has gone untouched by the disease.

Instead of taking an *HIV-first* perspective, which looks at the biomedical realities of HIV as it maps onto social life, I use what I call a *kinship-first* perspective throughout this book, a ground-up analysis that explores Basotho sociality—that malleable and fluid matrix where the people of Mokhotlong experience the disease most acutely and most personally. I see the social worlds of my interlocutors as the soil in which HIV/AIDS takes root, permanently altering the landscape. Yet it is the social world where people live and dwell. HIV is merely a part of the terrain. This kinship-first perspective will shed new light on ideas about Sesotho kinship, orphan care within families, and the ways that people understand HIV/AIDS.

While Basotho desire and strive for good health, their idea of health is deeply embedded in a relational view of the world. A biomedical understanding of the disease is not enough. Through the ethnographic data that animate these pages, with insights from medical anthropology and kinship scholarship, and with a critical eye toward structural inequality, I present people's experiences of living and caring in the midst of the pandemic. The AIDS that rural Basotho people know is a kinship disease.

## SITUATING AIDS IN LESOTHO

Lesotho is a small landlocked country that lies completely within South Africa's border, with a population of just over two million people. While surrounded by its larger and more prominent neighbor, it is geographically quite distinct. Crossing the border from South Africa into Lesotho, which sits on an elevated plateau, the landscape shifts immediately, with industrialized fields of maize replaced by more haphazard and varied family-owned farms. The capital city of Maseru, on the western border near Bloemfontein, has the feel of other small southern African capital cities. With a population of a quarter million, Maseru has a small business district of banks and government offices and a few newer malls where young urban elites and children in school uniforms gather for fast food and shop for the newest fashions and housewares. The city's bustling taxi stand is lined with rickety stalls selling fried dough balls (*makoenya*) and various grilled meats served with heaping domes of maize meal (*papa*). Some vendors offer socks and balaclavas for the cold winters. Indigenous healers lay out herbs, roots, and tinctures that people use to treat ailments as diverse as the common cold, chronic pain, and HIV itself. On the road leading out of Maseru, four lanes of dense traffic slim quickly into a two-lane country road where cars and taxis aggressively jockey with older pickups, swerving into oncoming traffic to gain position. This road leads past textile factories—largely run by Chinese businesses—and a handful of hotels where expats, visiting football teams, and government officials gather. Pope John Paul II Road lines the edge of a field where a large white tent and cross commemorate the Bishop of Rome's 1988 visit. Soon the city proper falls away, and communities of farms and villages and makeshift churches take hold over the red earth of the lowlands. Large newly built houses sit beside corrugated shacks, and the Maloti Mountains loom behind graveyards of car parts.

En route to the mountainous highlands, Teyateyaneng awaits: the district's central town, one of 10 regional hubs (or camptowns) that serve as administrative centers throughout the country. T.Y.—as Teyateyaneng is known in shorthand—is a third the size of Maseru and less than an hour's drive away. Up in Mokhotlong, people perform a dance move called T.Y., which entails turning around and going back where you came from—a joking commentary, it seems, on the highlands' perceived rural isolation and a sarcastic warning about what one should do when reaching Teyateyaneng, the point of no return, after which only endless rugged landscapes predominate. After T.Y., the district camptowns—home to government offices, large warehouses, hospitals, and police stations—decrease in size, especially in the highland districts. Beyond the rural villages of the foothills, the road into the mountains climbs sharply, winding along cliff edges, switchback after switchback, before plateauing in the heart of the mountain kingdom. For some time, the only signs of human habitation are mining vehicles, a ski hill with a lone broad slope, and groups of two and three shepherds leading sheep or cattle across rocky tundra. Depending on how recently the heavily pockmarked road has been repaired—suffering continual cycles of freeze and thaw—the next stretch of driving takes anywhere between two and four hours, passing one of Lesotho's large diamond mines and then dropping into the villages of Mokhotlong district, low enough for people to grow maize, wheat, sorghum, and a variety of root vegetables and leafy greens. Here, where the highway simply ends in Mokhotlong camptown, I lived at small local NGO called Mokhotlong Children's Services (MCS) and conducted over two years of ethnographic fieldwork between 2007 and 2015. Mokhotlong is home to around 13,000 people (Lesotho Bureau of Statistics 2016), a hospital, four high schools, a prison, a new grocery store, two hotels, a few NGOs, and scores of shops, shacks, and shanties, all tucked alongside the serpentine contours of the Senqu River.

Lesotho can feel remote and isolated, particularly in the highlands, where overland travel is onerous and where heavy winter snows occasionally make the roads impassable. But beyond its geography, the country's geopolitical positioning as an enclave has also had a drastic impact on its economic well-being and the progression of AIDS through its population. Lesotho is a poor nation (according to UN classifications, it is a least-developed country), and while literacy rates are high due to free primary education, 57 percent of the population lives below the poverty line because of limited opportunities for wage labor; in addition, food insecurity is routinely exacerbated by drought. Lesotho also has one of the shortest average life expectancies in the world—48 years—largely due to the spread of HIV (UNDP 2013). The first AIDS patient in Lesotho was an East African health worker who tested positive for the disease in 1986 (Government of Lesotho 2006), but it was not until the early 1990s that HIV began to spread in earnest, eventually reaching a stable adult prevalence rate of 23 percent near the end of the decade (UNAIDS 2010). The current adult HIV prevalence rate is estimated to be between 23 and 25 percent—a far cry from the "end of AIDS" discourse circulating among public health communities, donors, and governments (Kenworthy, Thomann, and Parker 2017). Lesotho's prevalence rate is surpassed only by Swaziland and Botswana, at 27 and 25 percent, respectively (UNAIDS 2014). Consequently, the average Mosotho[3] person can expect to live only into her late 40s, the same age as someone living in Lesotho in the 1960s.[4] But AIDS does not impact all age groups equally. Because most elderly Basotho were past their sexual prime when HIV started to spread in the 1990s, HIV is much less prevalent among the elderly than among other adult age groups, though older people living with HIV are steadily increasing in number as treatment has enabled people to live long enough to become grandparents.

What these statistics also mask is the unequal distribution of death and dependency that characterizes life for Basotho. Some people are infected; others are not. Some get tested in time and receive lifesaving drugs; others do not. Many die young; others are left behind to care for the increasing number of dependent adults and children left in death's wake. Infant mortality and under-five mortality rates are astonishingly high. But again, statistics about child mortality can eclipse rather than illuminate, masking the intense and often prolonged labor that goes into caring for a dying child. Despite concerted efforts by the government and numerous local and international NGOs working in the areas of prevention, testing, and treatment, the AIDS rate in Lesotho has essentially been stable for the past 15 years. Part of the ethnographic work of this book is to make these statistics real and palpable, replacing the figures with human experiences in their social context. An effective response to HIV depends on reading beyond the numbers.

Because the country is small, both in geographical size and population, there are far fewer individuals living with HIV in Lesotho than in countries with much lower prevalence rates. India, for example, has a 0.3 percent adult HIV prevalence rate, which translates to 2.1 million infected individuals, more than the entire population of Lesotho (UNAIDS 2017). Despite its small size, the dense and pervasive presence of AIDS in Lesotho makes it a relevant locale for studying the ways in which AIDS is embedded in communities and families. In a country like India, the impact of AIDS on families is far more diffuse and hidden. In Lesotho, with nearly a quarter of the adult population infected, no family has gone untouched by the disease.

Consider what it would mean if a quarter of your adult family members, your coworkers, your classmates, or your sexual partners were suffering from a deadly illness that was transmitted in highly intimate ways along social and familial lines. HIV in southern Africa and much of the Global South is far from the manageable chronic illness that it has become elsewhere, largely for structural reasons. While the first line of lifesaving antiretroviral drugs are readily available and free of charge across much of southern Africa, lack of personnel, the dearth of treatment options, generalized poverty, and structural barriers that hinder access, adherence, and support mean that AIDS has not abated. As many critical global health scholars have noted, not all lives are valued equally. Available treatments in the Global South lag behind treatments in the Global North by 20 years, despite there being appropriate health care delivery systems in place, often because the political will does not exist to spend the money that would save those lives. As Paul Farmer (2001) and others have noted, talking about "cost-effectiveness" becomes a dodge to avoid discussing the differential value of human lives.

Following critical medical anthropology, in this book, I take as the starting point a political economy of health perspective, which examines the economic and structural contexts in which health problems flourish (Baer, Singer, and Johnsen 1986). The laws, policies, and practices (biomedical and otherwise) that have facilitated the proliferation of AIDS in Lesotho cannot be separated from the global political-economic structures in which they have arisen. Tony McMichael, an Australian epidemiologist, wrote the most illuminating analogy on this concept that I have read, an explanation of the need to look at structures in order to understand a population's health. McMichael was critical of his own field for "explaining and quantifying the bobbing of corks on the surface waters, while largely disregarding the stronger undercurrents that determine where, on average, the cluster of corks ends up along the shoreline of risk" (1995, 634). These invisible "undercurrents" largely explain why so many corks—in this case, people living with HIV—have ended up on Lesotho's shores, and it is to these political-economic and structural factors that I now turn.

In Lesotho, a series of particular historical and political-economic conditions led to the rapid proliferation of HIV. Perhaps the most devastating was the small nation's geopolitical position as an enclave within South Africa and its economic reliance on migrant labor within the surrounding provinces. Basotho families have long depended on subsistence agriculture. Rural households typically own a number of fields where families grow staple grains such as maize, wheat, and sorghum. Residents of Mokhotlong also grow beans, peas, and potatoes in their family fields and cultivate cabbage, leafy greens, and root vegetables in the gardens adjacent to their houses. However, monocropping, overgrazing, soil exhaustion, severe erosion and land tenure disputes have forced many Basotho to seek employment elsewhere. In 1999, only 3 percent of Basotho farmers produced enough grain to live on, forcing men—and more recently, women—to seek work in neighboring South Africa (Coplan 2001).

Basotho men have been working in South African gold mines since the 1860s. By the late 1970s, 70 percent of the average Basotho household income came from migrant labor (Murray 1981). The chronic separation of Basotho men and women was necessitated by what Romero-Daza and Himmelgreen call Lesotho's "perpetual state of economic dependency" (1998, 200). It is no surprise, then, that decades of spousal separation had a significant impact on marriage, gender relations, and fatherhood. Anthropologists Colin Murray and David Coplan studied the impact of migrant labor on Basotho families over the last half of the 20th century, when apartheid laws did not allow women to join their husbands in the mining camps. Murray noted that "the enforced separation of spouses generate[d] acute anxiety, insecurity and conflict" (1981, 103). Despite that Basotho men spent 35 percent of their time in South African mines, Lesotho was where their "real lives" took place—or what Coplan calls their "socially significant and culturally meaningful existence" (1987, 419). In the mines, Coplan argues, men did not have any cultural authority, and upon returning home to Lesotho, they were determined to reassert it. The restrictive immigration laws made women at once dependent on men for cash but also gave them a degree of independence in their husbands' extended absences (Coplan 1987). Even once apartheid laws were lifted in 1994, many Basotho women chose not to join their spouses at the mining camps, as the living conditions were poor (Ramphele 1993), and many had familial and agricultural responsibilities that made relocation difficult. Once HIV began to spread in South Africa, migrant laborers were among the most vulnerable populations, contracting HIV from sex workers or long-term partners while away at work and spreading the virus to their spouses while on home visits (Romero-Daza and Himmelgreen 1998).

Male migrant labor to South Africa is no longer nearly as pervasive in Lesotho because of widespread mine closures and the fall of gold prices (Spiegel 1981; Lesotho Bureau of Statistics 2008). Yet opportunities for cash wages in Lesotho are still limited,[5] and Basotho frequently migrate to the lowlands of Lesotho or to South Africa in search of work. Increased female labor migration and rural-to-urban migration for a fluctuating textile industry continue to disrupt social life and increase Basotho's risk of exposure to HIV (Crush et al. 2010; Turkon et al. 2009; Coplan 2001). Among my own interlocutors, unemployment was high, and anxiety about finding work and money were frequent topics of discussion. However, the structural and geopolitical inequalities that continue to propel the spread of HIV also lead to poverty and unemployment and cannot be easily disentangled.

The HIV pandemic in Lesotho did not hinge on one infected doctor; in hindsight, rather, it seems a devastating confluence of events. Although migrant labor significantly reduced between 1996 and 2005, HIV continued to spread (Lesotho Bureau of Statistics 2008). In 1993, the HIV prevalence rate in Lesotho was approximately 5 percent—a high rate by any epidemic standard. By the late 1990s, the number had spiked to between 23 and 25 percent, where it has remained (Lesotho Ministry of Health 2016). Despite alarmingly high HIV rates as early as the mid-1990s, the government did not establish the Lesotho AIDS Programme Coordinating Authority until 2001, and it did not have a strategic plan in place, undertaken by the newly formed National AIDS Commission, until 2005 (WHO 2005). This late response to the pandemic took its cues from neighboring political and economic powerhouse South Africa, whose history with HIV is fraught with confusion, stigma, denial, and mismanagement by the government (Fassin 2007).[6] It was not long before the trickle of HIV that flowed from the mining camps in South Africa to the rural parts of Lesotho had grown to a steady stream. But soon, discussion of the original high-risk groups, such as miners and sex workers, became less germane as HIV was generalized into the population. When government officials finally rolled out the National AIDS Strategic Plan in 2005, treatment was not yet seen as a necessary element of the response (Government of Lesotho 2000; WHO 2005).

ART (antiretroviral therapy) was first available in Lesotho in 2002 at 2 urban hospitals. By 2005, 12 hospitals were offering ART; by 2009, more than 100 hospitals and clinics (both public and private) were offering free treatment (Owusu-Ampomah, Naysmith, and Rubincam 2009).[7] Despite this improvement, ART access remains well below the government target of 90 percent by 2020 (Lesotho Ministry of Health 2015). In 2005, only 13 percent of those in need of ART were receiving it. By 2016, this number rose to 53 percent for adults (UNAIDS 2017). In the early years of AIDS, a positive HIV test meant profound social shame, visible and rapid deterioration, and certain painful death. With this horrifying and dehumanizing outcome and no chance of treatment, it is not surprising that people avoided testing. But the widespread availability of ART in Lesotho has begun to show a significant impact in reducing AIDS-related deaths, which went from 15,000 people in 2005 to 9,900 people in 2016 (UNAIDS 2017). For children, maternal treatment means fewer orphans and lower rates of transmission from mother to child (Lesotho Ministry of Health 2010).

Health services for people living with HIV/AIDS in Lesotho are financed through a dizzying array of public and private funds. Between 2005 and 2008, almost 60 percent of funds for HIV/AIDS services came from international donors. Consequently, service delivery is inconsistent throughout the country, focused in urban centers, and susceptible to the volatility of the donors (Mwase et al. 2010).[8] Over the past few years, Lesotho has established a strong framework for HIV services: the government has developed policies and guidelines for a behavior-change communication strategy, a male circumcision policy, an antenatal-care registry, a childbirth registry, and revised guidelines for opportunistic infections like tuberculosis (TB). However, high demand has strained the country's capacity for delivering and ensuring the quality of these services (Mwase et al. 2010; Lesotho Ministry of Health 2015; see also chapter 2).

Despite significant improvements over the past decade, services for those living with HIV/AIDS in Lesotho remain limited. The country lacks the resources and personnel to deliver and implement existing policies. The confusing combination of grants, programs, and funding opportunities makes it difficult for patients and organizations alike to navigate the ever-changing terrain (Kenworthy 2017). These limitations mean that much-needed services—such as programs supporting caregivers for AIDS orphans or programs addressing the psychological impacts of AIDS—take a backseat to the more pressing needs of ART delivery.

## SITUATING AIDS IN A MOSOTHO

Most Americans who test positive for HIV will receive a battery of tests and surveys to assess viral load, CD4 count (cluster of differentiation 4, a measure of the body's immune response), general health, health behaviors, support systems, and readiness to begin treatment. These tests will help determine the antiretroviral treatment regimen that is most likely to work for a particular patient, with attention to health indicators (such as age, gender, liver function, etc.) and potential side effects. A patient's viral load is then retested every three to six months for drug resistance. If the virus is detectable, patients can switch to a new ART regimen. When starting on a three-drug (or combination) cocktail or when switching drug regimens, doctors and patients choose from a variety of antiretroviral drugs, which are optimized in various combinations of integrase strand transfer inhibitors, nonnucleoside reverse transcriptase inhibitors, nucleoside reverse transcriptase inhibitors, and protease inhibitors (HRSA 2014). A newly diagnosed 20-year-old living with HIV in the United States can expect to live into her early 70s (Samji et al. 2013). Once a harrowing death sentence that devastated the gay community in the 1980s, HIV is now a manageable chronic illness for most people living with the infection in the United States.

The contrast to Lesotho is stark. In order to test for HIV, first, one must go to the local hospital or clinic, often requiring a day's travel, or happen upon a community event with mobile testing capabilities. The WHO (World Health Organization) recommends that sexually active adults test for HIV every three months—the incubation period for HIV infection—because an HIV test would not detect the virus in a newly infected person. Yet in 2014, only 58 percent of women and 36 percent of men in Lesotho tested for HIV that entire year, a dramatic increase over previous years (Lesotho Ministry of Health 2016). At a hospital or clinic, a person trained in voluntary counseling and testing will use a finger prick (rapid test) to determine one's HIV status in a matter of minutes. If the result is positive, the patient must have blood drawn in order to test the CD4 count. Ideally, blood is drawn right away, but qualified personnel are in high demand and sometimes unavailable; other times, there is no vehicle to transport the blood to a lab. Or at times, the blood is successfully drawn and transported, only to arrive at a broken CD4 machine, where the sample is discarded untested. If a patient's CD4 count is less than 350 or if they are pregnant or less than one year old, they (or their caregiver) are required to attend three adherence sessions run by the ministry of health before they can receive the drugs. At these three sessions, where the same information is presented in triplicate, a patient (ideally, with a treatment supporter older than 12) will learn basic information about HIV, ART, side effects, proper nutrition, and opportunistic infections. Once the three sessions are completed and once the three confirming signatures are entered into their health booklet (*bukana*), only then can the patient begin treatment. In 2016, Lesotho launched a pilot program called "Test and Start," based on WHO recommendations that all patients who test positive for HIV start on the full course of ART immediately. This has yet to be rolled out nationally, but promising early results suggest that the country will move toward this practice as long as funding for the program remains in place (Schwitters 2017).

Deciding on a drug regimen might involve a quick assessment of suitability (such as an evaluation of potential side effects), associated testing (such as a pregnancy or liver-function test if supplies are available), and most importantly, the availability of the drug at that particular clinic (something that is never guaranteed). Each month, patients must line up at their clinic on an assigned day to check adherence (nurses count pills and log the results in a large government-issued ledger), discuss complications or opportunistic infections (if there is time), and then wait in line again for the pharmacist to refill their scripts and dispense their monthly medications. This takes a full day before the trip home, often on foot.

Currently, in Lesotho, only first-line antiretroviral drugs are readily available. If a patient is experiencing treatment failure (and it is recognized), a nurse or doctor can appeal to a medical board in Maseru to begin the much-more-expensive second line of ARV treatment, which is not yet available in a generic form as of this writing (February 2019). Because antiretroviral medication has only been widely available in Lesotho since 2004 (UNAIDS 2010), there are still few people in need of second-line treatment. However, access to generic second-line drugs will soon emerge as critical, given the challenges of good adherence in this rural context and given the natural life span of any line of treatment. With a lack of access to second-line drugs, treatment failure will invariably follow, greatly increasing the caregiving burden. I suspect that already, many of the cases I witnessed that were labelled "poor adherence" were in fact treatment failure, but neither the rural clinics nor the pharmacies were prepared to diagnose and treat for that.

While HIV destroys the immune response of any body it infects, regardless of race or nationality, an HIV diagnosis clearly means something different for a Mosotho than for an American. Understanding these differences demands a critical biocultural approach. Biological and medical anthropologists have long understood that human health is biocultural. As Leatherman and Goodman put it, "The many imbrications, linkages, and intersections between biology and culture . . . occupy a central place in medical anthropology" (2014, 29). In this context, a *critical* biocultural lens helps illuminate how political-economic, structural, and cultural forces shape people's experiences of health and illness. While I did not collect biospecimens or biometric data (except when reported by patients) as part of this research, I do consider the embodied experience of living with HIV and the differential biomedical outcomes—such as opportunistic infections and lowered life expectancy—that characterize the physical reality of HIV for my Basotho interlocutors and their caregivers.

Fortunately, in Lesotho, an HIV diagnosis is no longer an immediate death sentence. Consequently, Basotho are more willing to test and start treatment, disclose their status to their sexual partners and families, and share a meal with someone they know to be living with HIV. Yet treatment for HIV in Lesotho remains decades behind what it is in the Global North. Life expectancy provides a good proxy for this inequality, and Lesotho's is the ninth-lowest on the planet (Cohen et al. 2009; CIA 2017). There remain countless invisible barriers to the prevention, testing, and treatment of HIV in Lesotho. While orphan care is the primary focus of this book, the structural inequalities that shape the global risk of HIV infection inevitably inform the stories that fill these pages.

## WHY ORPHANS?

It seems almost banal to say that the high rate of HIV infection and the speed with which it spread have had a dramatic impact on Basotho families. AIDS is not only the major cause of death for the adult population; it is also the main cause of vulnerability for children left behind. In 2014, 27 percent of children under the age of 18 were single or double orphans, the majority of whom were orphaned because of AIDS (Lesotho Ministry of Health 2015). There are an estimated 78,000 AIDS orphans in Lesotho and between 1,500 and 2,000 new pediatric HIV cases each year (Lesotho Ministry of Health 2015).[9] These statistics obscure the depth and impact of this problem. Imagine being able to walk into any neighborhood in the United States and ask the first person you see, "Where are the orphans?" This is, more or less, how I often found families to talk to when I first arrived in a new village. While the pervasiveness of orphanhood made the recruitment of caregivers for this research easier, the experience was perpetually unsettling.

The analytic category of the orphan has been much debated. Scholars of AIDS orphans grapple with the "orphan" category because the existence of the category itself alters the material realities and kin relations of orphans. Cheney (2017) shows how development responses have reified orphans and vulnerable children as a category in need of identification and aid. Bianca Dahl (2014) powerfully demonstrates how, in Botswana and elsewhere, the category of orphan is locally constituted and mutable, and the aid provided to orphans is not always helpful, often alienating them from their families and setting them apart as "other." The orphan category is not merely pertinent as an item for scholarly debate, however; it has become a part of the development complex's response to orphaned children and, from there, has entered into the local lexicon as a means of accessing much-needed services. But the category of the orphan has its limits and can draw attention away from realities on the ground. According to Patricia Henderson (2011), the "African orphan" is imagined as existing outside of the family, destitute and alone. Yet I, like Henderson and many others, have found that most orphans are cared for by family members. As Jessaca Leinaweaver (2008) notes of Peruvian orphans, the socially significant orphan is not the child who has lost both parents but the one who has become socially detached. In Lesotho, all children—not just orphans—are made vulnerable not only by AIDS but also by poverty and structural inequality. Some orphaned children are better off than children whose parents are still living. Yet orphanhood brings with it significant challenges that are worth investigating. It is because of their real and imagined importance that AIDS orphans deserve analytical and ethnographic attention.

While the orphan-as-cultural-trope is relevant to the context of rural Mok-hotlong, where NGOs and government programs target orphans directly, the children who populate this ethnographic work experience orphanhood less as an identity category and more so as a material reality. For the children who I worked with, most less than five years old, the death of a parent—a mother in particular—had real and devastating consequences for their health and well-being, resulting in material deprivation and frequent caregiver changes. Throughout these pages, I aim to present a fully realized picture of the lives of orphans and their caregivers, demonstrating that orphans are not living outside the fold of family but struggling alongside their families in complex mutual relations of care.

Fleshing out the lived experiences of orphans is crucial because in rural southern Africa, AIDS has dramatically affected orphan care and altered the structure and makeup of the family. In Lesotho, people have strong extended family ties, which help ensure that children are cared for in times of need. However, kinship networks that previously protected children from orphanhood often become overwhelmed due to HIV-related illness and death (Townsend and Dawes 2004; Heymann and Kidman 2009). The AIDS pandemic serves as the disheartening backdrop for the physical, material, and emotional challenges of orphan care and the reorganization of families. And while these changes have wider roots and resonances, the prism of orphan care offers an opportunity to explore them.

Orphan care is illuminating because patrilineality is rooted in reproduction (children), and Basotho responses to the orphan crisis underscore the deep connections between HIV and kinship. Children are the focal point of marriage and are key to social reproduction.[10] Bridewealth, a cultural practice that is tied to customary marriage, involves the payment from the groom's family to the bride's family of an agreed-upon number of livestock (or its cash equivalent). Though a declining practice, bridewealth remains symbolically significant for securing the lineality of children who belong to the patriline if bridewealth has been paid (Block 2014). Families invest in their sons' children with the hope that they will inherit fields and homes, care for them when they are old, carry on the family name and clan, and continue to connect generations of ancestors through ritual feasts. As a result, children are highly valued and cared for even in times of duress (see chapter 1). Basotho society has always been organized to allow for the shared care of children through extensive fostering systems. AIDS has disrupted, though not destroyed, these fostering networks. Changing practices around orphan care highlight the flexibility of kinship as it is deployed to care for its most vulnerable members.

Orphanhood is also a revealing lens for HIV's impact on caregiving practices, due to both the affective dimensions of Basotho child care and its dura-
tion. The care of children, particularly young children and those living with HIV,
is labor intensive and highly visible to outsiders like me. Care of sick adults is
recondite and frequently involves the kind of stigma that prevents it from occurring openly (consider the difference between bathing a sick child and bathing
a sick adult). The sheer visibility makes the caregiving practices for orphaned
children a potent site for analysis. Basotho children are also dependent on adults
for many years, providing ample time to observe care practices and shifting kin
bonds. The vast majority of children I began working with in 2007 were less than
five years old at the time. The longitudinal nature of this eight-year study has provided powerful insight into their growth, their joys and successes, and in some
sad cases, their deaths and the deaths of their caregivers.

Orphan care rearranges families and households, as I illustrate, pushing
the boundaries of lineality and other idealized markers of relatedness as a response
to the sheer scale of circulating orphans in the AIDS era. As an extensive body of
research has shown, this care is still almost exclusively taken on by family members (Adato et al. 2005; Ansell and van Blerk 2004; Cooper 2012; Nyambedha,
Wandibba, and Aagaard-Hansen 2003; Prazak 2012; Zagheni 2011). Parents and
caregivers have reimagined the place of children within families, as they move
from household to household in sometimes unexpected ways, given the strength
of patrilineal norms in Lesotho. One of the most significant findings of my
research is that Basotho privilege care over many other things. Once they find a
suitable caregiver for a child, they decide how to create a narrative around that
caregiver that fits with dominant patrilineal and patriarchal norms. Caregiving
networks are under strain in part because HIV has permeated kinship—but the
primacy of care means that many children could be much worse off than
they are.

The ways that children—orphans in particular—are cared for in Lesotho
are changing. Yet these contemporary care practices are situated within a complex social and biocultural environment. The structure of this book builds
toward an examination of the matrilocal care of AIDS orphans, first laying a
conceptual foundation and then proceeding through layered ideas that illuminate the changing process. I begin this book with a look at kinship practices
broadly—fundamental for understanding contemporary orphan care and the
changing kinship landscape (chapter 1). I then consider the different ways that
Basotho think about health and illness generally and HIV specifically (chapters 2 and 3). With this cultural context established, I address the evolving ways
AIDS orphans are cared for in the midst of a pandemic that has been altering and
undermining the fabric of social life in Lesotho for decades (chapter 4), examining AIDS as a kinship disease through the lens of orphan care. While the first

three body chapters lay the groundwork for the theoretical argument that comes in chapter 4, the ethnographic material throughout the book is largely drawn from the experiences of orphans and their caregivers.

## RELATIONALITY AND CARE IN PRACTICE

A few months before I first left for the field as a graduate student in 2007, I completed my comprehensive exams. I remember lugging a large rolling suitcase full of African ethnographies and theory books across the campus and back to the library. I thought myself well informed at the time. When I arrived in Lesotho, I embarked upon my fieldwork on the lookout for what these books emphasized was a decidedly African "relational" view of the world—or what John and Jean Comaroff refer to in Tswana personhood as an "intrinsically social construction" (2001, 268). In Mokhotlong, I inquired about the naming practices of children and noted how married women changed their names to "mother of" their child's name, reflecting this relational view of the world and emphasizing the importance of procreation. And I noticed how people repeatedly asked me about my own children (nonexistent at the time), who they assumed I had left at home with a grandmother while I worked in Lesotho.

After a few months, I met an American couple who worked and lived in the lowlands and were caring for four orphaned Basotho children less than two years old. In each of the four cases, the child's primary caregiver had passed away, and the extended family members had refused to take the child in, either due to a lack of ability or lack of desire to care for them. After the American couple had been living with the children for six months, they sought to legally adopt them and obtain passports so they could bring them back to the United States. The adoption process, however, necessitated that each Mosotho family sign a letter saying they were transferring all rights and responsibilities to the American couple. Although none of the extended family members had visited any of the children during that period, and while all of the extended family members had declared themselves unwilling or unable to care for the children, three of the four families refused to sign the letters. These families would have been content to have the American couple live with the children, but the concept of permanently signing away the children was incoherent within the local system of child fostering, which works to maintain—not sever—ties between kin. This experience devastated the American couple, who had difficulty comprehending the Basotho families' objections, since they had never displayed any kind of overt affection, emotional connection, or even physical proximity to the children. It revealed to me that I needed to think carefully about what this relational view of the world meant to people's ideas of family and how a strong sense of kinship might not necessarily involve affective signifiers of love or care. I began to investigate how relationality and care overlapped and diverged and what that meant for both kinship and relatedness.

This book rests its foundation on a theory of practice, whereby people's actions and negotiations around the care of orphans are more powerful than the "official" story they tell about who is supposed to care for orphans. As Bourdieu notes, this approach privileges kin relations that are "continuously practiced, kept up, and cultivated" through everyday actions, rather than those that are upheld as the "official" way things should be done (1977, 37). In practice, according to Bourdieu, rules may not be desirable and therefore may not be followed. Sherry Ortner, who expanded and built on the work of Bourdieu and others, notes that while there have been many developments in practice theory, most scholars agree that action is not "sheer en-actment or execution of rules as norms" (1984, 150). In other words, people have never simply followed rules because they are there, but rules and norms are reinforced by "highly patterned and routinized behavior in systemic reproduction" (Ortner 1984, 150). In this book, I look at the changes in patterns of orphan care as a response to HIV/AIDS and how they differ from the stated norms and rules that Basotho report about kinship, which (as Ortner and others agree) have always been at odds. The gap between the stated rules and lived realities tells us where practice differs from, as Geertz famously phrased it, "the stories we tell ourselves about ourselves" (Geertz 1973, 448).

Once I started investigating how and why people care for children, particularly orphans, I found ready evidence of a widespread system of fostering that has survived even in the face of major economic and social disruption. Fostering allows for the temporary and flexible movement of children between households and helps maintain kinship ties through shared lived experiences. Yet emerging patterns of fostering do not conform to Basotho people's idealized versions of their strongly patrilineal and patrilocal society. Patrilineality in Lesotho manifests itself in a number of ways. It is an ideology that shapes interactions between clan members and affines (in-laws) through naming practices, monikers, and appropriate signs of deference and respect. In more practical terms, it has a number of real-world impacts. It presupposes that a young mother will go to her in-laws if she needs to borrow food or money (a privilege that comes with paid bridewealth); that children will only inherit from their father's family, with sons dividing up houses and fields when the older generation dies; and that orphans will be cared for by a paternal relative, preferably their father's mother. In reality, household arrangements, inheritance, and care are far more varied, even while names and clans remain strongly patrilineal. In the ever-growing space between the ideal and the real, the distinction between "kinship" and "relatedness" is experienced by Mokhotlong residents. This is most evident in the ways that people care for orphans.

The distinction between kinship and relatedness stems from the 1970s and 1980s, when scholars launched a critical salvo against old-guard anthropological theories concerning kin relations. Thus kinship scholarship no longer relies on its original foundations, which tied it closely to biology and genealogy (Peletz 1995). Largely driven by feminist scholars, the concept of kinship has become decoupled from nature. This has meant that a single theory of kinship can no longer encompass all possible family forms, opening up the possibility for new relationships that were previously excluded from the list of one's kin. Some results of this shift include moving away from an assumption of heteronormative family forms (Weston 1991); questioning "natural" bonds, such as that between a mother and child (Holý 1996); and analyzing the dissolution of ties that were once assumed to be indissoluble (Biehl 2005; Borneman 1997). In order to express this new "broad and imaginative view of what might be included under the rubric of 'kinship,'" Carsten proposes the use of the term *relatedness* in order to "signal an openness to indigenous idioms of being related rather than a reliance on pre-given definitions or previous revisions" (2000, 4). While Basotho kinship ideals are still important, bonds formed through everyday practices of care are what shape relatedness—or kinship in practice.

Basotho still identify strongly as patrilineal; in theory, descent is traced through the father's family. However, kin relations have changed due to a number of historical, political-economic, and demographic pressures—AIDS is only the most recent. Long before AIDS, as already noted, generations of Basotho men spent the better part of their adult lives working in the gold mines of South Africa, leaving behind "gold widows"—women who saw their husbands for only a few months a year and, in their absences, took on the responsibility of heads of their households, in charge of their families and fields. As a result, some of the practices most closely associated with patrilineality—marriage, bridewealth payments, and a fostering system that highly values patrilocal coresidence—have declined, even as patrilineal ideals persist. While these idealized notions of patrilineality are still important in understanding Basotho kinship, patterns and practices of care, especially for orphans, are increasingly relevant to understanding everyday experiences of relatedness. In other words, the intimate acts involved in caring for a young child are fundamental to the affective bonds being formed. These bonds are part of the complicated web of kin relations to which Basotho still strongly ascribe, but they have a force and power of their own that stems from shared spaces, shared substances, and shared daily experiences of joy and suffering.

A relational view of the world encompasses both idealized kinship and everyday caregiving practices. Later in the book, I will devote considerable attention to caregiving processes as they manifest in this context. In Lesotho, care has emerged as the strongest motivation for new patterns of social organization.

Increasingly, the willingness to care, as demonstrated by everyday acts of caring, has become most important in influencing patterns of child fostering. Over time, caregiving practices that have arisen during the AIDS pandemic have begun to shift even firmly held idealized notions of what family means to the people of Mokhotlong.

## COMPLICATING AIDS AS A KINSHIP DISEASE

During my fieldwork, people often told me that the biggest problem they faced was AIDS. This was rather memorably expressed to me by 77-year-old 'M'e Mapoloko, who attributed all her problems to HIV, despite her age and the fact that her husband had died more than 20 years prior. One day, while she was casually lamenting her various ailments, from itchy armpits to a sore back, she said, "I think it is [HIV]. Because everyone can be suffering from it. If you are suffering from the nose or the ears, they are now itching—you are having HIV." When I reminded her that most cases of adult HIV in Lesotho were sexually transmitted, she laughed and said, "I don't know if I have got it some years ago," implying delicately that she had not been sexually active for some time.

In some ways, this overemphasis on AIDS is understandable. No other issue has had the broad impact on adult and child mortality and on changing networks of care throughout this country. And yet Basotho families face myriad other pressures, from a chronic shortage of available jobs, to poor access to basic health care, to a host of medical maladies beyond AIDS. Noncommunicable diseases such as respiratory infections, cardiovascular disease, cancer, and diabetes account for 27 percent of all deaths in Lesotho (WHO 2014). What I aim to show here is not simply that AIDS is different from other illnesses in how it moves socially through communities but that by integrating biosocial and relational approaches, we can learn much about how any illness moves through communities—a process informative not only for infectious diseases of epic proportions but for many other social ailments as well.

Let me return briefly to Matseli, the young boy whose story opened this chapter, who succumbed to diarrheal disease on the way to the clinic, despite adhering to his ARVs and notwithstanding the love and good care of his maternal grandparents. Matseli had AIDS. AIDS compromised his immune system, weakened his heart, and prevented his small body from fighting the infection that took him so quickly. Yet his story exemplifies the multivalent complexity of AIDS, from how the disease alters social life in ways that go beyond the sick individual to the distal and murky structural factors that produce conditions where AIDS thrives. Matseli contracted HIV through his mother, a woman whose marriage was weakened by migrant labor—a practice fundamentally connected to Lesotho's geopolitical position as an enclave within South Africa and a practice that has been impacted by, among other things: apartheid, the extraction of gold, the sudden appearance of textile factories in the lowlands, and the soil erosion that makes subsistence agriculture all but impossible. Matseli's inability to get treatment during the Easter holiday goes beyond the missionary spread of Christianity (but is not completely divorced from it) to the unequal spread of the disease and available treatments globally. His story touches on the ways that AIDS reverberates through kinship, changing people's understanding of the disease and altering social networks to address the needs of orphans. Like many Basotho, Matseli's grandmother, 'M'e Maliehi, told me that she thought AIDS was a "disease like any other"—a position that allows families to raise HIV-infected children with an eye toward their future, investing in their education and hoping they will be able to live a normal life. This relational understanding led to 'M'e Maliehi's surprise at her grandson's sudden death, since he was not displaying outward symptoms of AIDS. Kinship allowed 'M'e Maliehi to care for her grandchildren, despite her tenuous position in their lineage due to the partial bridewealth paid at the time of her daughter's marriage. And kinship led Matseli to be buried with his father's kin, despite their apparent indifference to him and his mother.

The social reality of orphan care is especially powerful in revealing AIDS as a kinship disease. When orphans are infected by HIV, they simultaneously present a serious caregiving challenge, one that threatens the social fabric of everyday life. Orphanhood invites reflection on the breakdown of marriage, the role of bridewealth in defining the bounds of family, the changing nature of gendered relationships, and the structural inequalities that have devastated many Basotho families. My hope is that a kinship-first view of AIDS will illuminate pathways that can alleviate the suffering of those infected and impacted by the disease.

## CONDUCTING FIELDWORK IN RURAL LESOTHO

Fieldwork in the remote rural highlands of Lesotho presents numerous challenges that surely are not unique in ethnographic research. But because they are unique to this book and greatly shape both what was possible for me and what my interlocutors experienced, I explore some of them here. I began my research with a preliminary two-month trip to the field in 2007, conducted a year of fieldwork from 2008 to 2009, then returned for two- and six-month stays in 2013 and 2015, respectively. Will and I lived on the grounds of Mokhotlong Children's Services, a small local NGO that serves orphans and vulnerable children. MCS was initially founded in 2004 by a graduated Peace Corps volunteer and his girlfriend (now wife). In 2005, they turned the leadership of the organization over to 'M'e Nthabiseng Lelimo, who has been the managing director ever since. After our first short visit in 2007, Will and I had a small rondavel[11] built on the grounds of the safe home, which now houses volunteers and medical personnel. I developed a close friendship and trusting work relationship with 'M'e Nthabiseng, whose son, Tumo, later came to live with us in the United States, first in 2013, during his gap year before starting college in South Africa and again in 2017, during a multimonth break from university.

Over the past 15 years, MCS has received funding from a combination of personal donations raised mostly through its U.S.-based foundation, from U.S.-based churches, and from institutional grants, including those from UNICEF (United Nations Children's Fund), Care, Sentebale (Prince Harry's Lesotho-based charity), and a German NGO that supports agricultural and environmental projects. MCS is the only organization providing comprehensive services to AIDS orphans and their families across the Mokhotlong district, with a population of approximately 100,000 (Lesotho Bureau of Statistics 2016). Although families receive some assistance through local clinics, hospitals, and other small NGOs, MCS is the only organization in this region that offers limited residential care for the most vulnerable children under five, makes home visits, and provides support to caregivers; thus it is the only program to reach the most remote and isolated communities. Because of this, MCS was an excellent place to begin my research. Although fieldwork in the mountains of Mokhotlong was challenging, I was able to observe the organization's service delivery for several months before branching out on my own, which significantly aided my work and local cultural knowledge.

To facilitate my entry into Basotho homes and to help with my budding Sesotho, I employed a research assistant, Ausi (or "sister") Ntsoaki Lerotholi, who translated during interviews and assisted in transcribing afterwards.[12] She generally made my research easier by helping accelerate my cultural learning, making sure I did not overstep my boundaries, and ensuring that I did not get lost on the many nameless paths I had to travel. She was my constant companion and became my dear friend. After I left Mokhotlong in 2009, Ausi Ntsoaki was hired by MCS, where she still works, so I had to find other research assistants on subsequent trips—usually through 'M'e Nthabiseng, who is well connected in Mokhotlong.

Our two eldest children were born in 2010 and 2012 and accompanied us on subsequent trips to Lesotho. Having them along helped me forge deep personal connections with my interlocutors. During their first trip (in 2013), my daughter, Eve, was only 10 months old and still breastfeeding. Most days, I strapped her to my back and took her with me to visit rural villages, often nursing her while I spent time with my friends. Children who saw us arrive would come to play with her, and if she was in the mood, they would take her around the village. Once I was done with my visit, I would wander around until I found Eve, who was often playing on the ground, surrounded by a group of friendly and curious children, or happily strapped to a young girl's back with a blanket and a large diaper pin. Once, I returned to find her dressed in another child's *seshoeshoe* dress—a formal piece of indigenous Sesotho clothing. While Mokhotlong hosts the occasional foreign tourist or NGO worker, I never saw another white child in the district until 2013, when an American missionary family moved into town. Bringing my children was both convenient for me and methodologically useful, as my interlocutors saw me perform the daily acts of care that they had not previously seen a white woman do. My friends were happy that I had become a mother, since childbearing is an important social marker of full womanhood in Mokhotlong. For better or for worse, I believe their respect for me grew when I returned to Lesotho with my children.

The geography of Lesotho—with limited and often impassable roads, severe soil erosion, and the occasional hard winter snowstorm—greatly hinders freedom of movement. Transit between Mokhotlong's outlying villages and the district's central camptown can range from a several-hour walk or taxi ride to a full day of travel in one direction. Due to the geographic isolation of the outlying villages, I bought a motorcycle during my longest stint (from 2008 to 2009), which allowed me to travel on both rugged paths and paved roads. On subsequent trips, when I often brought one or both of my children with me to the villages, I hired a car. Many of my fieldwork destinations required both a drive and a hike. Although I attempted to cluster visits in the same general direction, I would often spend several hours trekking toward one caregiver, only to find them away at the clinic, working in the fields, or elsewhere. When I first started my fieldwork, it was nearly impossible to schedule visits because phone service and the electricity or batteries required to charge mobile phones were spotty at best, and instead of making appointments to visit people, I would just drop by. If we were expecting a call from our families in North America, Will and I would usually climb up the mountain behind MCS to get better reception. Over the past decade, cell service has improved, and most rural families own a mobile phone for use when they come into town, which they charge in the village with an old car battery. Most younger interlocutors and MCS employees living in town have internet-enabled mobile phones and communicate regularly with family and friends living elsewhere in Lesotho and abroad. By 2015, most older caregivers and those living in rural areas at least had access to a simple mobile phone. I now communicate regularly with my friends in Lesotho on Facebook and WhatsApp, a popular communication tool used widely outside the United States, which allows users to make affordable voice and video calls, send pictures, and leave lengthy voice messages for friends and family abroad.

When Ausi Ntsoaki and I traveled between villages during my yearlong stay, people were at first puzzled to find two young women riding around on a small dirt bike. A few other NGOs in the area had motorcycles, including Riders for

Health, a group that delivers supplies to rural clinics and transports blood samples to the lab at the hospital. However, I only saw a few per week, driven exclusively by men. The sight of our bobbing red helmets quickly became familiar, though, and those expecting us would keep an eye out for our "horse," as one grandmother told me. Apart from taxi drivers, few rural residents in Mokhotlong own vehicles, and many of the families I worked with did not have the disposable income to pay for regular transportation. The challenges I experienced in accessing the villages and homes of caregivers are exponentially greater for the caregivers themselves.

To get around in Mokhotlong, people often travel in notoriously crowded minibus taxis, which drive along the main road and down some of the dirt tracks that branch toward rural villages. Once, while traveling to South Africa by minibus, we watched the small-statured driver of our vehicle let a larger man take the wheel while he, the original driver, hopped onto the dashboard facing the front-seat passenger—all to create space so that one more rider could squeeze into the minibus. On another occasion, our driver stopped an already-full minibus taxi to pick up a mother and two children. The woman passed her baby to Will and—with her older child on her lap—wedged into the middle bench beside him. Once situated, however, she did not take the baby back—so densely were we packed into that vehicle—but instead pulled out her breast and nursed the baby in Will's arms while we traveled. In the Mokhotlong camptown itself, there are numerous four-plus-ones (standard taxis) that honk up and down the main strip, taking people from one end of town to the other or to any number of drop-off points along the main highway. Many people forego taxis, though, and simply walk or ride their horses or donkeys into town. Beasts of burden, saddled with children or enormous sacks of maize en route to the community mill, are frequent sights along the road. And for most, a trip into town takes a full day. To get to Maseru from Mokhotlong, one can take a series of minibus taxis through several drop-off zones; there is also a large coach bus that leaves early in the morning and arrives eight hours later. No matter the mode of transportation, schedules are fluid, and patience is cultivated quickly.

The distance between my field sites and the difficulty of travel did not always permit me to spend long stretches of time with my interlocutors. I would often enjoy an hour or two of conversation with someone and then continue on to visit another family nearby or make the long journey home. This painstaking and time-consuming method of data collection was not efficient, but it was the best way to gain insight into the lives of rural Basotho that more convenient methods of data collection—such as working with patients at a clinic or in villages close to town—would not allow. Throughout this book, I focus on the interviews and conversations I had with people, as well as my own observations, resulting in an unconventional "commuter" ethnography that has its limitations. Yet I believe the insights here are conveyed most powerfully by privileging the voices and words of Basotho caregivers, and throughout these pages, I leave in their verbal musings, their uncertainties, and the idiosyncrasies of their speech so that the reader can understand and interpret the evidence in context.

The content of my conversations was often highly sensitive. To address this challenge, as noted, I observed service delivery with MCS outreach workers for several months before starting a new series of visits to the caregivers on my own. This allowed me to build rapport with potential interlocutors and to increase my understanding of problems on the ground before delving into questions of a sensitive nature. I visited caregivers at least twice with MCS prior to visiting them with only my research assistant, Ausi Ntsoaki. I then began a series of interviews, visiting every few weeks, starting with the most general and least personal material. I also spent time during each visit chatting informally with caregivers and playing with the children, in order to directly observe care and increase the comfort level of the caregivers. I made additional casual visits with Will and, since 2013, with our children, sometimes for special celebrations or events. By the time we talked about sensitive issues, such as HIV and the challenges of care, we had been acquainted for the better part of a year and had built a trusting relationship. I became close with many of these caregivers, and they often used kin terms to refer to me (*ngoaneso*, which means "my sister/sibling" or, more colloquially, "my dear"). They also used kin terms regarding the bond I shared with the children in their care—referring to me as the child's "mother" or to them as my "children." This, of course, comes with its own complex set of racial and power dynamics, which I address below. But I believe their thoughtful, honest, and personal responses reflect genuine closeness.

This book is dominated by the voices of women, many elderly. For the most part, this is because Basotho women continue to provide the majority of care for orphans and sick family members, adding to what Henderson calls the "structural marginalization" of women, of which caregiving duties are only one dimension (2011, 177). Ethnographic work on caregiving such as this also gives a voice to women who have been historically marginalized in the public realm, whose labors are often not recorded or recounted. However, the male voices presented here indicate that much could be gained from understanding male perspectives on care and that men are increasingly important as caregivers as the demographic pressures of AIDS and the demands of an increasingly feminized migrant-labor economy create shortages among family caregivers.

A primary challenge of the interpretive task in ethnographic research is to write about people's recollections of times and events. I often explicitly asked my interlocutors to think about their current circumstances by reflecting on the past, but people often brought up experiences and memories without my prompting. Because many caregivers I spoke with were elderly, their memories often went back years, sometimes decades. Throughout the book, I represent people's memories as just that: reflections on previous events or experiences as seen through their present lens. I am not attempting to write an ethnography, for example, about what life was like for migrant laborers and their families in the 1970s. These have already been written by people working during that era (see, for example, Murray 1981; Coplan 1987). Rather, I am curious how people's perceptions of the past influence their experiences of the present. For example, I want to know how the familial disruption caused by migrant labor—which I learned about through ethnographic research and literature reviews—alters people's experiences of the changes HIV/AIDS has brought to family life. As noted previously, I start from the premise that cultural ideals are rarely closely followed in practice. Thus when caregivers lamented the failure of families to adhere to ideals of orphan care, it was important to me not whether those ideals were *actually* practiced in the past and are no longer but that caregivers *thought* those ideals were practiced and that they are still upheld as the gold standard in orphan care. I start from the assumption that my interlocutors' memories are more likely to be romanticized in contrast with the present—or as Boyer and Wertsch argue, such memories are "idealized, simplified representations" of cultural scripts (2009, 31). Or perhaps, as the historian Pierre Nora suggests, the mere passage of time causes disequilibrium, due to the nature of "an increasingly rapid slippage of the present into a historical past that is gone for good, a general perception that anything and everything may disappear" (1989, 7). Finally, wherever possible, I compare people's ideas about social change (as when people claim that there are more orphans nowadays) with contemporary data (which widely acknowledge that this is true), in order to get a sense of how life truly has changed for caregivers and orphans in Mokhotlong.

As is often the case, anthropologists become entangled in their field sites in ways that are both rewarding and problematic. We find ourselves involved in intimate personal relationships and friendships that open doors for us ethnographically yet put us in compromised positions in terms of what we write, who we have access to, and what unseen alliances we make—sometimes inadvertently—that shape and structure the types of knowledge we gain. Thus it is necessary for me to say a few more words about Mokhotlong, my connection to MCS, and my position in the community. It did not occur to me until I took my first trip into South Africa how different the racial tensions and perceptions of foreigners (*makhooa*)[13] were in Lesotho, as compared with its powerful surrounding neighbor. Interactions between whites and blacks become palpably charged as you drive across the border into the Free State, toward Bloemfontein, where Afrikaans-speaking white South Africans are clustered. There are also numerous overt signs of government influence and wealth. The cracked ochre earth of Lesotho is almost immediately replaced by large expanses of green, with herds of fattened cattle grazing inside vast fenced areas. This obvious wealth brings with it predictable disparities in South Africa: shantytowns outside urban areas and, in the cities, beggars and street children coexisting uncomfortably alongside luxury cars and houses with elaborate security fences. In rather striking contrast, 75 percent of Lesotho's population lives in rural areas, and over 99 percent of the population is ethnic Basotho, contributing to reduced racial and ethnic tensions and a more generalized distribution of poverty (Mwase et al. 2010; WHO 2005). While Lesotho's rural areas lack South Africa's wealth, they also lack the obvious disparities and ongoing racial tensions that are a pervasive legacy of the apartheid state. Lesotho is almost entirely culturally and linguistically homogeneous. Apart from a few Xhosa villages near the South African border, a small but visible number of Chinese merchants and shop owners, and a small population of foreign Africans (mostly nurses, doctors, and businessmen, referred to derisively as *makoerekoere*[14]), Lesotho consists predominantly of Sesotho-speaking Basotho people.

Maseru is the locus of many NGO headquarters, and while it is not uncommon to see white Europeans and North Americans in the capital, this diversity does not extend to the mountain district of Mokhotlong. In Mokhotlong, attitudes toward foreigners ranged from curiosity and interest to indifference. Because there are no white Basotho and the majority of the population is geographically isolated, the most devastating effects of apartheid on rural Lesotho appear in the political-economic realm—and yet the political-economic and social realms are intimately linked. The social implications of structural violence caused by apartheid and its oppressive policies during the period of intense labor migration have greatly affected Basotho people. Nowhere is this truer than the impact of HIV/AIDS on the family.

The generally positive prevailing Basotho attitudes about white foreigners certainly eased my fieldwork experience. However, this ease makes reflexivity (because of my position as a white, educated, and wealthy foreign woman) even more important. Among my more mortifying experiences during fieldwork were the numerous occasions when 'M'e Nthabiseng, MCS's managing director, sent me to collect medications for MCS clients, instructing me to skip the hours-long queue for the pharmacy. MCS had good reason to do this: because they care for so many babies, they would need a full-time employee just to wait in line at the hospital for lifesaving medicine, where a villager or caregiver might only have to come to the hospital for this experience once a month or less. Yet it was not merely a matter of convenience that 'M'e Nthabiseng sent the predominantly white foreigners to do this unpleasant task. She was well aware of the authority that whiteness and foreigners carry, particularly at the hospital, where foreign staff and volunteers are frequently encountered. People waiting to pick up medicine would likely yell at a Mosotho employee of MCS who attempted to skip the queue, as I often saw happen to other Basotho line-skippers, but this never happened to me. Despite my efforts to treat people with respect and kindness and to privilege local perspectives and ways of knowing, power differences are stark and unavoidable. My position as a white foreigner greatly impacted my interactions with people, and to the best of my ability, I tried to ensure that consent to participate in my research was truly voluntary.

My alliance with MCS benefited me both socially and professionally. In addition to observing service delivery through MCS, I was connected with caregivers and orphans in the outlying villages. Living at the safe home also situated me at a locus of activities; as the only residential care facility for orphans in the district, I witnessed many cases unfold, particularly emergencies, as caregivers brought children to MCS in desperate hope of receiving assistance. Clients and potential clients constantly stopped by to ask questions or to collect medications and supplies. The proximity, both geographically and professionally, of MCS to the district hospital also increased my familiarity with happenings there. I was often asked to take children to the hospital, bring supplies to clients, or check on potential clients there. I got to know the non-Basotho African doctors (mostly Zimbabwean and Congolese) and the American doctors and had the opportunity to observe service delivery, accompanying doctors and nurses on rounds and taking children to appointments.

However, my relationship with MCS was also fundamentally collaborative. Although I most often did my work in the villages while Will taught at the local public high school, the staff viewed us as long-term volunteers, frequently asking us to help with various chores or with the babies in the safe home. In addition to daily assistance in and around MCS, I helped implement an improved data-collection system for MCS that involved months of work. I helped design and test the database, trained outreach workers on data collection and data entry, and entered much of the preliminary data myself. I first met most of the caregivers I worked with through MCS; therefore, my role was initially confusing to them, since they saw me as a part of the organization. This was exacerbated by the fact that I often delivered food or messages for MCS when I was traveling to a village to do interviews in order to save outreach workers an entire day of work and fuel expenses. Although I have no medical training, I quickly learned a great deal about HIV treatment, preventing malnutrition and dehydration, and recognizing the symptoms of opportunistic infections. At the request of MCS, when visiting a family whose child was HIV positive, I often began by looking at their health booklet (*bukana*) and medication supply to ensure that they would not run out before their next scheduled visit (which was sometimes the case). I was also asked to make sure that caregivers were properly administering the complicated and frequently changing medications. I found many instances where the clinic had made errors in scheduling the next appointment or where the care-giver was giving a child an incorrect dose. Given the importance of adherence to ARVs, I continued this practice throughout my time there. I would also look through health booklets to make sure that a child's HIV testing was up to date, since young children require a complex system of retesting to confirm their HIV status. This was often neglected by the overworked and underresourced clinic and hospital staff, and to ensure that these errors were remedied, I occasionally recorded necessary information in the health booklets to alert health care pro-viders of the child's needs. I felt obligated to perform these simple and important checks, which at times had life-or-death implications for children I knew well. They were also educational for me in learning about the challenges of care for HIV-positive children and the failures of the health system.

In some ways, my connections to MCS and my involvement in monitoring the health and well-being of the children complicated my role as a researcher. My interlocutors often assumed that I had some authority as a health care provider. Although I never attempted to give this impression and repeatedly explained my role to people, this misconception was difficult to dispel, especially for care-givers who knew me through MCS. However, through long-term engagement in the field site, through my ability to measure caregiver self-reporting against what I observed over time, and through my own reflexivity and awareness of potential biases and power imbalances, I attempted to remediate these complicating fac-tors and so minimize the pitfalls associated with the nature of my relationship with caregivers. It is my sincere belief that even as caregivers saw me as a poten-tial resource, the amount of time we spent together allowed me to obtain hon-est and important information about kinship and care. While my relationship with MCS created some challenges, it also provided opportunities for me and gave me insight into the community in ways that would not have been available otherwise.

## CHAPTER OVERVIEW

As the concept of relatedness is central to orphan care and since I am arguing that a kinship-first perspective brings new and important insights to a well-explored topic, I begin with kinship. Chapter 1, "Kinship First," examines what it means to be a Mosotho. I investigate how people live, with whom they live, and how kin ties are made and unmade. In these examples, I demonstrate that while Basotho ideals about kinship are based on the principles of patrilineality, relatedness is formed, maintained, and dissolved through the practices of living—particularly caregiving. I focus here on conceptions of relatedness, with an emphasis on memories and practices around caregiving and the importance of houses and house life. Through the process of remembering, elderly caregivers first articulate their broader concerns about the changing nature of kinship and social life.

In chapter 2, "Medical Pluralism in a Low-Resource Setting," I show how Basotho's treatment-seeking decisions are localized, culturally produced responses to poverty and structural inequality. Mokhotlong residents seek solutions to their health problems from both biomedical doctors and indigenous healers not merely in response to cultural beliefs and practices but because of the globally unequal distribution of health care resources and personnel. Yet both because of and in spite of the structural constraints on treatment seeking, people in Mokhotlong continue to make decisions that protect their social relations. While therapies, policies, and resources shift, families remain ever present—even as they adapt. These beliefs and behaviors set the stage for Basotho responses to HIV treatment, testing, and prevention efforts and reinforce the importance of kin in addressing health problems.

In chapter 3, "Like Any Other Disease," using the critical lens of medical anthropology and focusing on knowledge and treatment, I explore the challenges of treating HIV/AIDS. While showing the extent to which social and familial concerns dictate and shape the pathology of the illness, I explore the significant structural barriers that impede treatment and prevention efforts and examine the role that stigma plays in shaping the epidemic. This investigation demonstrates the real challenges of AIDS, particularly for the care of orphans.

The book culminates in the findings of chapter 4, "Orphan Care and the Family," where I show how AIDS intersects with care to shape community responses to the "orphan problem" in Lesotho. My ethnographic examples illustrate Basotho ideas of caregiving, with reference to the widespread practice of kin-based fostering. I illustrate how cultural ideals about gender are not fixed but rather flexible cultural constructs that can be deployed to privilege orphan care. There has been a gradual shift toward increasing care by maternal relatives, and while Basotho have maintained an ideal of patrilineality, paradoxically, they explain this matrilocal care largely by invoking the rules of patrilineal descent.

Finally, in the conclusion, "Infected Kin," I summarize the practical and theoretical contributions of this book and demonstrate their applicability to orphan care more broadly. Focusing on the importance of understanding that AIDS is a kinship disease, in how the disease itself infects and changes networks of kin and as a proxy for making sense of the less tangible historical, structural, and political-economic influences, I illustrate the changed nature of sociality in southern Africa. I conclude by looking ahead to one of the most pressing questions facing Basotho society today: what impact will grandmaternal mortality have on families as the AIDS pandemic continues to burn through southern Africa?

As with this introduction, each of the following chapters begins with a literary nonfiction vignette written by Will McGrath, writing he produced by fusing his own observations and experiences (since many of these families he has known for years) with my field notes, transcripts, and photographs. The main body of each chapter is the work of the ethnographer (Block), and any errors or omissions are my own.

# 1 · KINSHIP FIRST

## In the House of 'M'e Masekha

*Once upon a time, there was a house.*

*This house was up in the eastern mountains of Lesotho, out past St. James, where the gorge is strung with power lines, delicate filaments that stitch together two halves of the earth. The lines are decorated with white and red plastic balls that hang at intervals like Chinese paper lanterns, a warning to low-flying aircraft, of which there are none.*

*The house was a rondavel, a small circular oasis that kept cool in the summer and held warmth deep into winter. Its wind-smoothed walls were made of piled rock, plastered with a paste of mud and dung, and its roof was smoke-darkened thatch. The earthen floor was smooth and cool, swept daily. A rondavel is circular because a circle is the best shape to absorb the strange branching energies of a family, and a family is an idea that forks and zags and curls back on itself.*

*Over the course of many years, this house bore witness to births and deaths and all the other circles and loops that occur in a lifetime. People left and got married and divorced and returned. Some were carried to the house in sickness and walked away in health. People left to find work or returned to find work or left and never returned. All the multicolored bonds of family were made and unmade inside the crucible of this house. When there were births, the men cleared far away, and a reed was placed over the door to notify people that this place was now private. The women scrubbed the smooth floor and cooked roots and bark to help the mother with her labor, and when the baby came, the mother washed her breast and fed it. After three days, the house was cleaned again, the blood and afterbirth covered over with a new layer of earthen plaster. In this way, all the important substances came together in the house and became a part of the house—milk and blood and food and medicine.*

*It was the same for death: a layer of sand was spread across the floor, and the body was undressed and cleaned and then dressed again in light clothing. After the burial, everyone returned to the village to share meat and joala.*

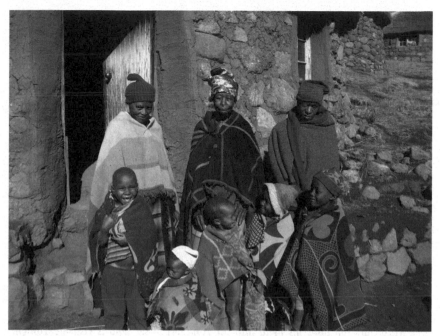

FIGURE 1.1. 'M'e Masekha (back center), Thapo (front left), and their family in front of 'M'e Masekha's home, Mokhotlong, 2009

*All of this took place inside the house. It was 'M'e Masekha's house, but it could have been anyone's.*

\* \* \*

*'M'e Masekha first came to this house from her parents' place when she got married. She had a husband, in a way.*

*At the time, there was no work in Lesotho, so her husband went off to the mines in Gauteng, South Africa. He worked there for 30 years like this: gone for a year, home for a month, gone for a year, home for a month. "It was difficult," 'M'e Masekha says, "but there was no other way. We didn't have money for some things—no one to help plow the fields." And there were other difficulties too—girlfriends that her husband had on the side. "We had our problems. I was talking to him about these girlfriends, but I stayed. People now are quick to divorce before they solve their problems."*

*After three decades of work, her husband came home from the mines and died. 'M'e Masekha taught preschool after he was gone, but that work dried up. She sold joala, got piecework jobs from neighbors, collected and sold wood, and sometimes worked on road construction crews. "But the ground is so hard now," she says. "I can't dig anymore—I don't have the energy." When she was desperate, the neighbors gave her* food, but everyone was desperate at some point, so she was careful not to depend on such kindnesses.

'M'e Masekha has children—three boys and two girls—but her girls died in their adulthood. "I am left with sons," she says, glancing quickly out the window. There are children playing outside, and for a moment, maybe she hopes to see her sons. But one is working in South Africa, and one is in Lesotho, down in the lowlands in Hlotse, selling cassettes at a stand in the market, that place where the taxis pull in and send a gentle dusting of red earth over the scores of gospel and famo tapes, even tapes by Barry White and Moikaele Mojakisane, which is the name that people use for Michael Jackson.

Her third son lives nearby in the village with his wife, but his two children live in 'M'e Masekha's house. There are four small children living with her currently, and sometimes there are five. Are these children siblings? Cousins? Ache—these distinctions become slippery—sometimes 'M'e Masekha calls them all her children, sometimes she calls them by their proper names, sometimes she uses more rigid genealogical distinctions. But they are all bound together in this house, where they share food, where they curl up together at night, snug on their sleeping mats on the smooth, cool floor.

* * *

'M'e Masekha's son pops his head into the rondavel to see who is visiting. Tonight, he and his wife will eat with 'M'e Masekha, as they do from time to time. The wife will breastfeed their daughter, one and a half years old now, before leaving the girl overnight. This granddaughter insists on sleeping with 'M'e Masekha often, and sometimes—'M'e Masekha is laughing now—sometimes the girl tries to pull on her breast in the night; even in sleep, even from her grandmother, the girl is seeking milk. Perhaps later other grandchildren will come to eat there too, older ones, the children of her son who works in South Africa. They come by frequently to help nkhono with chores, playing with the smaller children or going off to gather wood and collect water from the tap.

Certainly, though, it is Thapo, of all her grandchildren, for whom 'M'e Masekha has carried the most responsibility. Thapo is 10 and has lived with 'M'e Masekha for several years now. He is the son of 'M'e Masekha's other deceased daughter, a woman who divorced her husband and returned to the village. The paternal side paid no bridewealth, and so they had no claim on Thapo.

When Thapo and his mother arrived in the village, they were both very sick. 'M'e Masekha spent several long days caring for them in her house: the three of them shared the small room while Thapo's mother cycled through bouts of vomiting and diarrhea. Soon 'M'e Masekha had them both in nappies. "I was changing the mother, then changing the baby, changing the baby, then changing the mother," she says. She bathed them and cared for them, her daughter and her grandson, and during those few days, the years looped back on themselves and blurred. "Thapo's mother was very sick," 'M'e Masekha says, "and she died because no one could help me take her to the doctors."

But Thapo has thrived under his grandmother's care. "Kannete, I'm happy," she says. "I was not expecting him to survive. He was not looking like a person. I couldn't wash him in front of other people—I was afraid to take his clothes off in front of others. But I was patient."

Thapo is big now, HIV positive but healthy, and he has learned how to manage his ARVs (antiretroviral drugs) well. He helps 'M'e Masekha around the house, doting on her earnestly, then checks the clock and takes his meds, then runs to fetch water. Now he slips quietly into the rondavel—school is done for the year—and places his report card on the table.

"Hele!" 'M'e Masekha shouts when she sees it. "This one is so clever. He is always coming first at school!" Thapo flushes with pride and simultaneously with shame—that complex dual emotion honed and perfected by young boys.

"Kannete, he is brilliant!" 'M'e Masekha says, brandishing the report card, and Thapo's only option is to flee the rondavel entirely.

\* \* \*

'M'e Masekha's family morphs and adapts, bouncing its strange energies off the circular walls of the rondavel. She remains close with her deceased husband's brother in the village, who comes to eat with her sometimes. She calls him a blood relative, although he is not, yet her own children she does not consider to be blood relatives. They are bonded by a more precious substance—bonded by milk.

Men, women, and children pass fluidly through the house, driven by an array of shifting pressures: economic, cultural, marital, material, and medical. Occasionally, people die and even then refuse to leave her house. "My father died in my hands," she says, "and my mother-in-law. And my husband died while I was sitting with him. When his soul went out, I saw it. And even now we dream about the people who have died, and we cook food for them and brew joala when they are absent." Even the ancestors can spare a moment now and then to share a meal with the living—even they have relationships that can be sustained through food and drink.

'M'e Masekha stops talking for a moment and looks around the rondavel. "Even my husband, I'm always dreaming about him, every time. I dream that I can see him."

\* \* \*

Once upon a time, there was a house, a rondavel up in the mountains, out where the gorge is knitted with power lines. Out there the hawks glide along thermals, circling and wheeling in endless frictionless loops, and a house is a circle too, which is the best shape for a family, and a family is just an idea.

-WM-

\* \* \*

## WHAT BINDS PEOPLE: KINSHIP, CAREGIVING, AND RELATEDNESS

As I embarked on this ethnographic project, I frequently encountered situations where my interlocutors would talk to me about how things should be done and then turn around and do something entirely different. A mother would tell me that her children should live with their father's family, and then she would send them to live with her own mother. A grandfather would tell me that women are to care for children, and then he would dutifully cook *papa* and *moroho* for his orphaned grandchildren and take them to the clinic each month for their checkups. As I started thinking about these "exceptions" in the aggregate, I began to notice what they all had in common: a compulsion to care. While AIDS is perhaps the motivating force that pushes webs of caregiving relations to the fore, this book is more about care and its consequences than it is about AIDS. The increased need for care and the resulting acts of caregiving (for orphans, for adults living with HIV, and for the elderly) are rewriting the rules of kinship and relatedness.

'M'e Masekha's caregiving story is a typical one in rural Lesotho; it represents the complex interconnections and relationships—and the associated life stories, joys, and struggles—that make up many households. When one steps back from the details of 'M'e Masekha's life, her experiences reinforce the notion that kinship is inherently flexible, even—or perhaps especially—when under immense pressure. This flexibility allows families to adapt to circumstances external to the family, both by bending the idealized rules of social relations and by rewriting them. In Lesotho, many factors are changing people's ideas about lineality—most obviously migrant labor and HIV/AIDS but also technology and education. Everyday life has become more difficult for rural Basotho because of HIV/AIDS and poverty, so it is not surprising that rural residents have begun to move away from some of the restrictive practices of a strongly patrilineal society, such as bridewealth payment and the patrilocal care of orphans. Yet my interlocutors' commitment and ability to care for children within the family—as opposed to orphanages or nonkin fostering—have remained strong. Under the strain of AIDS and high rates of orphaning, care has become the primary organizing principle of social life. The locus of that care is increasingly centered on the house, making coresidence more important in shaping relatedness.

Networks of extended kin in Lesotho are central to rearing and caring for children. For example, nearly 500 children were cared for in the MCS (Mokhotlong Children's Services) safe home between 2005 and 2018, yet only five ended up in the care of nonkin—two in an orphanage in Maseru, two children with special needs in residential facilities in the lowlands, and one adopted by an American couple. Children are often raised by a number of different caregivers for various practical, social, and material reasons. These fostering networks, which have a lengthy history in Lesotho and elsewhere in Africa, Latin America, and Oceania, are impacted by the nature of kinship ties and are subject to change as the needs and practices of communities evolve. Therefore, understanding the context of contemporary Basotho kinship beliefs and practices is central to understanding kin-based care for orphans.

Many of my elderly interlocutors expressed the concern that family life is more unstable now than in the past, when filial responsibility was taken more seriously, family ties were stronger, and the income generated by migrant labor in South Africa made life easier. The conversations in this chapter are based on my interlocutors' ideas about kinship ties and family responsibility, as well as ethnographic observations about everyday life. However, there is likely a considerable gap between memory and reality, especially when it comes to remembering or forgetting the social and marital disruption caused by migrant labor that spanned the better part of a century (Murray 1981; 1976). Still, Basotho ideas and experiences regarding relationships between family members, the makeup of households, and kinship and family responsibility are real and relevant. Their expectations highlight the complex nature of social organization and the disconnect between the ideal family structure (patrilineality) and everyday practice. In what follows, I address these aspects of relatedness—both real and idealized—that are key to the ways that kinship ties are created and dissolved. Through this ethnographic exploration, I lay the groundwork for examining the importance of the Sesotho house. I present a picture of an institution and space that plays a central role in the everyday life of Basotho families, where relatedness is shaped by the increased importance of coresidence in the time of AIDS care. Finally, I consider the impact these multiple factors have on orphan care.

## CARE AS PRACTICE

As the anthropologist Julie Livingston put it, "Caregiving is a moral endeavor" (Livingston 2012, 96). The moral nature of care, about which much has been written (see, for example, Kleinman 2012; Mol 2008), is complicated by the physical and social disruption of HIV/AIDS in Lesotho. This book is dominated by what Annemarie Mol (2008) calls "a logic of care," in which care is central to practice and is a social and moral good. Care is, according to Mol (2008, 75), a "crucial moral act," one that values attentiveness and specificity, eschews neglect, and aims to make life better for people. Yet because care is complex and is different across space and time, there is no clear path or set of rules that can establish what "good" care looks like (Mol, Moser, and Pols 2010). Instead, good care emerges through practice. As Arthur Kleinman so eloquently wrote while reflecting upon the loving care he provided for his wife, who was suffering from

Alzheimer's, "It is a practice of empathic imagination, responsibility, witnessing, and solidarity with those in great need" (2009, 293). Because of the extremely personal nature of caregiving and because caregiving in much of the world is done by family members—especially women—care and kinship are deeply intertwined (Manderson and Block 2016). Yet while the best care might be tied to affection, this coupling between care and love should not be assumed to be natural. The possibility that care and love might not operate in tandem gives weight to the moral nature of caregiving and ties it inexorably to kinship.

AIDS-related care brings these affective assumptions and the flexibility of kin relations into sharp relief. In Lesotho, as elsewhere in southern Africa, kin relations cannot prescribe or predict who will take on the labor of care (Manderson, Block, and Mkhwanazi 2016). Caregiving is subject to the vagaries of chance, geography, access to resources, affection, and relatedness (Merten 2016; Nxumalo, Goudge, and Manderson 2016). People—represented here and across the caregiving literature—use different strategies to protect their caregiving relationships, building up "care capital" (Manderson, Block, and Mkhwanazi 2016, 4), which can be cashed in at some future time when the caregiver herself may be in need of care. The motivations, economic conditions, and material and affective realities of care in the time of AIDS differ greatly, giving further weight to the need for a practice approach to understanding care and its consequences in the context of HIV/AIDS in Lesotho.

## WHAT'S IN A NAME?

Patrilineality remains a pervasive cultural ideal among Basotho. It is a powerful ideology that orients people to their living kin and ancestral lineages. Lineality is one of many modes of reckoning kinship, as expressed through kin terms, names, clans, and places of origin. These terms and names reinforce the importance of lineality and are used as a way of showing respect, honor, and social position within the family. But while patrilineal ideals remain important as anchors of moral geography and kinship, the social indicators of the *practice* of patrilineality—such as inheritance and kin terms—are more varied. Like all idealizations of culture, lineality has never been static or strictly followed (Bohannan 1952), but in Lesotho, changes in practice seem to have been accelerated by migrant labor, evolving marriage patterns, and the demographic shifts caused by HIV/AIDS. Thus patrilineality is often far more important as a cultural ideal than in the practice of everyday living and caring.

In Sesotho culture, a woman marries into her husband's family and takes his name, though she remains part of her natal (birth) clan. Even among families who adhere to these patrilineal practices, women and children continue to have important relationships with their maternal kin, but these relationships emphasize social interactions over material ones. Children take their father's name and clan and belong to their father's family, particularly if bridewealth has been paid, and in theory, children inherit land from their fathers, and their fathers' families are responsible for their upbringing and education. Recent legal advances in Lesotho have removed the minority status of women and protected their rights to property and custody of their children.[1] But while customary law, which favors sons, can no longer be upheld by civil courts, it is still frequently invoked in resolving disputes at the local level. While the Lesotho Land Regulations from 2011 do not specify inheritance only by paternal relatives, matrilineal land inheritance is far less common in practice (Sekatle 2011). Yet 'M'e Nthabiseng believes that women are increasingly inheriting property from both sides of the family. "It's slowly being practiced," she told me, "because now people decide to give their properties to their favorite kids or kids who actually provide for the family." Thus idealized rules of patrilineality are superseded by the need for willing and able caregivers.

Ancestry is another way of maintaining patrilineal kin ties and highlights the potency of lineality as a cultural ideal. 'M'e Mamorena, an elderly caregiver of two paternal great-granddaughters, invoked the disapproval of her ancestors to affirm the importance of following Sesotho rules (meaning patrilineal rules): "Sesotho rules are difficult. In Sesotho rules, when there are orphans, they should go to the father's side, because when the mother wakes up where she is buried, she will just come straight to my house, not to her home, and say she wants her children. And she will be asking, 'M'e, where are my children? Have you lost them?' And she will not go to her [natal] home. She will just come here." For 'M'e Mamorena, care, ancestry, and lineality are connected and confirmed by her own situation as a caregiver of paternal orphans. If these grandchildren had been her maternal kin, she would likely have answered this question in a way that justified her care of them. By using the term *Sesotho rules*, 'M'e Mamorena subtly acknowledges that Sesotho culture and practice are not one and the same, just as someone might point to an "official policy." Drawing attention to the "officialness" of certain rules implies that there are unofficial ones that guide people as well. My interlocutors' frequent references to "Sesotho rules" both confirm the continued importance of idealized notions of patrilineality and reveal the unofficial rules that guide behavior.

The terms used to delineate kin are important because they not only reflect but also help reproduce social relationships (Radcliffe-Brown and Forde 1951). Kin terms used by Basotho to identify their relatives are partially unilineal—there are some different terms for relatives on the paternal and maternal sides of the family—and they indicate the importance of maintaining lineal distinctions and the significance of relative age. There are specific names to indicate if an aunt or uncle is on the mother's side or the father's side and names to indicate a younger sibling instead of an older one. These are not used exclusively, as people will often default to generic kin terms such as *ausi* (sister) or *abuti* (brother), but they are used when distinction is deemed necessary. But not all Sesotho kin terms are unilineal. A person would use the word *ngoaneso* (my sibling) to refer to one's mother's sisters' children or one's father's brothers' children and the word *motsoala* (cousin) to refer to one's mother's brothers' children or one's father's sisters' children. In other words, parents' same-sex siblings' children are called "siblings," but parents' opposite-sex siblings' children are called "cousins." In practice, the closeness of the relationship between these unilineally differenti-ated cousins is based on other social factors, such as proximity. There are also terms such as *grandmother, grandfather*, and *grandchild* that are not differentiated on the basis of lineage.

Sesotho honorifics, which translate into kin terms, are used habitually. The most commonly used honorifics translate into the words *mother* ('m'e), *father* (*ntate*), *sister* (*ausi*), *brother* (*abuti*), *grandmother* (*nkhono*), and *grandfather* (*ntate-moholo*). Even close friends and relatives call each other 'm'e or *ntate*, followed by their given names. In addressing strangers, one must also choose an honorific most closely associated with age and stage of life. When trying to decipher kin networks, the term of respect used for someone does not necessarily indicate his or her specific relationship, thus elaboration is often necessary. For example, when I asked one caregiver about her relationship to the child in her care, she said, "Mamokete is the child of my *molamo*. . . . It's the child of the sister of my husband." In this case, she used the term *molamo*, which means sibling-in-law, but she had to explain this further to distinguish between a sister-in-law and a brother-in-law. When Basotho describe their kin, they often have extremely complicated and contextualized ways of describing their relationships to each other. When I asked 'M'e Maliapeng, a 47-year-old caregiver of two orphans, how she was related to someone, she replied, "When he sees the grandmother, the mother of my father-in-law, he is saying *rakhali* [father's sister]." In this way, she used a kin term to note the nature of their relatedness (by marriage) and also indicate the generation to which the relative belongs. Further, age brings with it important status for Basotho; using the terms for grandmother (*nkhono*) and grandfather (*ntate-moholo*) is extremely important among family and strang-ers alike. The speaker's specific relationship to the older person is often unclear, since an older aunt, uncle, or even sibling could be called *nkhono* or *ntate-moholo*. For example, children address their mother's older sisters as *nkhono*, yet they call their mother's younger sisters *mangoane*. Those caregivers I got to know well were aware of my interest in kinship and the nature of relationships and were often explicit in describing their relations and the kin terms they were using. It was at times like these that I was most thankful for my digital voice recorder.

Basotho inheritance rules and kin terms help maintain a unilineal system by distinguishing between the maternal and paternal sides of the family. The perseverance of unilineal kin terms helps reinforce the ideal of patrilineality, even though in practice, orphans are often cared for by their maternal kin. In some ways, the obfuscation of genealogical relations embedded in both kin terms and the local parlance reflects the fact that specification is often not relevant to Basotho. During the time of AIDS, patrilineality has become secondary in maintaining strong ties to family members. Instead, a sense of responsibility and obligation to kin is now held together by such conditions as proximity, cohabitation, reciprocal aid, love, health, and the capacity to help. The flexibility and widespread usage of more general kin terms may help legitimize caregiver-orphan relationships that do not fit into the idealized patterns of care and make room for the affective bonds that shape Basotho families into less predictable configurations.

## MARRIAGE IN FLUX

Attitudes about love and emotion are not natural but are embedded in cultural institutions such as marriage and its correlated social divisions—natal kin (relatives by birth) and affinal kin (relatives by marriage). Changes in marriage across sub-Saharan Africa are difficult to measure because of the variation across the region, the increase in informal unions, the uneven reporting of state and customary marriages and divorces, and the processual nature of marriage, which makes marital status more difficult to pinpoint at any given moment. There has been a decline in marriage rates in Lesotho over the last 50 years: in 1989, 70 percent of Basotho women were married by the age of 25, and 95 percent by the age of 30 (Timaeus and Graham 1989), but in the past three Lesotho Ministry of Health demographic health surveys (from 2004, 2009, and 2014), one-third of women of childbearing age had never married. Although, in many sub-Saharan African countries, remarriage is more common than remaining uncoupled after the dissolution of a marriage or widowhood, in Lesotho and other countries with high HIV prevalence rates, formerly married men and women are likely to remain unmarried (de Walque and Kline 2012). One reason may be because remarried men and women are more likely to be living with HIV than those who are unmarried or in their first marriage (Ramashwar 2012). While my interlocutors sometimes articulated HIV risk as a reason for remaining single, more often than not, they expressed that they had tried marriage, and it had failed them, so they did not feel the need to try it again. Perhaps this is why many women I spoke with felt that divorce was more common now than in the past, even though divorce rates have remained relatively stable according to the last three demographic health surveys (around 5 percent to 7 percent for women and 3 percent to 5 percent for men).

But while marriage ideals have remained fairly stable, marriage patterns and family life have changed, first significantly in the 1970s due to migrant labor (Timaeus and Graham 1989; Murray 1981) and since the 1990s because of HIV/AIDS. My interlocutors in Mokhotlong, both young and old, acutely felt that marriage was different than it was in the imagined past, and these differences impacted women's relationships with their natal and affinal kin and changed how children were cared for within the extended family. The slow changes in marriage and divorce mask the acute anxiety and discomfort that rural Basotho feel about the disconnect between marital ideals and the lived reality of their relationships.

## THE PHYSIOLOGY OF KINSHIP

For Basotho men, fatherhood marks the transition from boy (*abuti*) to man (*ntate*). Yet the idealized importance of patrilineality—of which procreation is a necessary part—is not primarily about biological relationships—it is a social theory of descent. The clearest evidence of the social emphasis on lineality is the distinction that Basotho make between *pater* (social father) and *genitor* (biological father). Perhaps the most famous African example of this comes from Evans-Pritchard's ethnography of the Nuer (1940), where through "ghost marriage," a widow can have children with another man (either her husband's brother or a different lover) who are deemed to belong to her deceased husband. The underlying purpose is to keep intact the patrilineal structure of the family and to make sure that the ownership of the cattle exchanged at the time of marriage remains clear. Rural Basotho, like the Nuer, at times de-emphasize biological fatherhood in favor of maintaining clear relationships and social positions within the family.

Although it is more frequent for the *pater* and *genitor* to be the same person, in many instances during my fieldwork, it became apparent that this was not the case. The selective de-emphasis on paternal biology is an important strategy used by caregivers to legitimize their role in the life of an orphan. For example, 'M'e Mamorena is the great-grandmother of three orphaned sisters, the youngest of whom, Hopolang, was a client of MCS. They are the children of 'M'e Mamorena's grandson. When MCS outreach workers were filling out the intake forms for Hopolang, 'M'e Mamorena listed under "father" the name of her grandson. However, after learning more about the family, I discovered that Hopolang was born several years after her "father" had left for South Africa and not returned. 'M'e Mamorena revealed that it had been years since she had seen her grandson: "In the past! *Hele*! A long time ago! He left her when she had two children, when she was breastfeeding that one [pointing to her middle great-granddaughter]. And the husband left the wife for a long time, and we don't know whether he is still alive or not. This wife had the child while she was not living with the husband."

I naively asked if Hopolang knew her father—thinking I might discover who the "real" father was. However, this did not register with 'M'e Mamorena, as the question was not relevant. Instead, she told me that even Hopolang's older sister did not know their father (meaning her grandson). Although I did not ask, given the tight-knit nature of the community, it is likely that 'M'e Mamorena knew the biological father's identity. But because she was a paternal great-grandmother and was responsible for caring for Hopolang, the question was irrelevant and might have challenged her position as caregiver. In another instance, six-year-old Rethabile was cared for by her *pater*—her mother's husband—after her mother's death. Her mother, however, had lived in South Africa for four years before Rethabile was born. Rethabile's *pater* could not possibly have been her biological father; he didn't meet her until she was almost two years old, when she returned from South Africa, critically ill with full-blown AIDS and TB (tuberculosis) and motherless. Nonetheless, he accepted her as his daughter and continued to take excellent care of her, despite his advanced age and her complex health needs. For these children, their places in the family were more important than their actual biological relationships to their fathers. Potential familial instability was avoided by de-emphasizing biology in favor of social security and mutual responsibility.

Kinship and lineality are fundamentally about sociality, and amid the AIDS pandemic, the lack of emphasis on biology works to protect orphans from abandonment. However, this should not imply that biology is irrelevant. Many Basotho held strong ideas about the importance of kin as opposed to nonkin, even as blood relations were symbolically salient rather than biologically important. The most compelling evidence for the ongoing importance of biological relations revolves around the care of children, who in rural areas, are still cared for almost exclusively by kin. Among rural Basotho, biology can be de-emphasized by decoupling *pater* and *genitor*, and biological ties—while important—are inherently flexible. In this context, caregiving relations and household makeup worked around the strict dictates of lineality.

## REPRODUCING KIN

During my fieldwork, people who knew that I was married and of childbearing age never asked me, "Do you have children?" but posed the question assumptively: "Where are your children?" or "How many children do you have?" When I did return to Mokhotlong with my own two young children in 2013, all my friends and acquaintances—especially the grandmothers—were thrilled and visibly relieved. Many made gifts to my children, including 'M'e Matau, who gave my daughter, Eve, a chicken (figure 1.2), and 'M'e Ithumeleng, an MCS staff

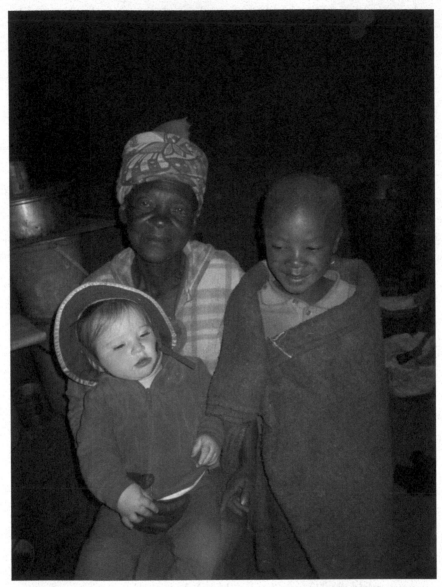

FIGURE 1.2. 'M'e Matau and Tsepi with Ellen and Will's daughter, Eve, in their home, Mokhotlong, 2013

member, who knitted my son, Sam, a hat embroidered with his Sesotho name, Samuele (figure 1.3). My friends' enthusiastic reception of my children reflects that the birth of a child is a celebrated event, despite an overall decrease in fertility in southern Africa and in Lesotho in particular.[2] Just as fatherhood is the mark of manhood for Basotho men, motherhood marks a girl's transition from *ausi* (sister) to *'m'e* (mother). For men, this transition reinforces ideals about lineality. For women, the importance of childbearing is focused on the embodied change in the woman, a metamorphosis that takes shape through pregnancy, labor, and the mother-child bond. Ideally, when a baby is born, the mother and child stay inside their house for up to three months to allow the mother to heal and to keep the child from ingesting harmful substances outside the home. During these months, only close male relatives are allowed to visit; the house is dominated by women who help the new mother with cooking, cleaning, and the care of her other children. The increase in orphans and the reduction of available and healthy caregivers have lessened neither the importance of children for Basotho nor the loving care I witnessed between many women in Mokhotlong and the babies in their homes.

The adaptive strategies used by Basotho to cope with the pressures of AIDS emphasize the well-being of orphaned children and ensure that care is primarily

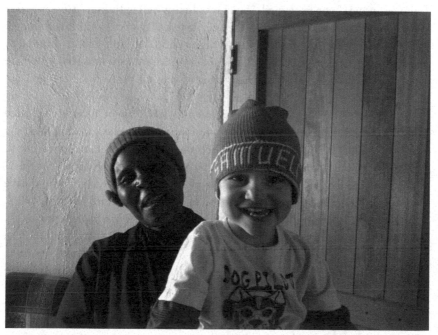

FIGURE 1.3. 'M'e Ithumeleng with Ellen and Will's son, Sam, wearing the hat she knitted for him, Mokhotlong, 2013

family based; they do not minimize the importance of children. Although a few older caregivers said women should not have children before marriage, more said that women should not get married (because they will end up divorced) and instead just raise children at their natal homes. 'M'e Maliapeng was 47 and a widow, and although married for many years, she and her husband had been unable to conceive. When her husband died, she was left at his family's village, childless and HIV positive. I chatted with her about her husband one sunny winter day as we sat outside her tidy square house while she prepared sorghum to brew *joala*. She told me that she wished she had never gotten married: "*Ache*,[3] I just think it's better for the girl to stay at her home because marriage has changed. It's no longer the same as in the past. . . . I just, see, if I was not married, maybe I was going to live in a good way at my home, maybe with my parents. It's so difficult in marriage, and life is not easy. . . . Even if she can have children, it's OK. But she should stay with the parents." I was surprised by this: 'M'e Maliapeng had openly talked about her husband with affection, lovingly showing me the house he had built her before he died and describing how he had been devoted to her despite their infertility and the tension this caused with her in-laws. While she admitted that her husband badly wanted children and took her to the doctor to try to solve what he assumed were her fertility issues, he was kind to her and refused to remarry despite his family's encouragement. "*Ache*, it is other people [who are cruel]," she explained, "but I was living well with him." However, fertility is a crucial consideration in the marriageability of a partner. A friend of Will's who taught with him at the local high school told him that he wanted to sleep with his wife before they got married to make sure she was fertile, but she would not let him. By protecting her virginity, she was protecting her marriageability as well.

Childbearing is considered a fundamental function of marriage (Pearce 1995). When I first met 'M'e Mamorena, Hopolang's great-grandmother, she was surprised by my upbeat attitude, which she assumed was incompatible with childlessness: "Why don't you have children, yet you are always happy like this?" I informed her that I wanted to complete my schooling first, and I would have them when I returned home. This seemed to satisfy and amuse her a great deal, as she replied, "Heee, ha! Okay, ha! *Kannete* [I swear]. Oh, *ngoaneso* [my dear]. Ah! My friend." Likely, she was amused by the nonsensical behavior of a *lekhooa* ("white person" or "foreigner," pl. *makhooa*). She told me that when I returned, I should bring my children so that she could watch them for me. Will was also asked occasionally by his colleagues if he had any children, particularly once they knew he was married. However, Basotho men commonly marry younger women, so a childless man in his late 20s was not as unusual as a childless woman of the same age. Once, when a male outreach worker found out that I was a year older than Will, he replied with some embarrassment, "Oh, in Lesotho, that is not ideal!"

The importance of children is reflected in the continued use of teknonyms among Basotho[4]—the practice where a woman changes her name after her first child to "mother of [child's name]." It is more common to name a mother after a male child, but both male and female teknonyms are used. For example, an outreach worker at MCS was named Karabo by her parents, but after the birth of her first child, Bokang, she changed her name to 'M'e Mabokang (mother of Bokang). After the birth of my son, Sam, in 2010, 'M'e Nthabiseng began addressing me in email exchanges—only half-jokingly—as 'M'e MaSam. This naming practice not only reinforces the importance of motherhood in Lesotho but also reflects the "socially embedded view of the self" that pervades Basotho identities (Gergen 1991, 7; Guma 2001).

Basotho names, taken from the Sesotho lexicon, are seldom chosen randomly (Ashton 1967). Children are frequently named after grandparents or great-grandparents, linking them to their ancestry. It is common to name a child after a positive characteristic or attribute because Basotho believe that a name will influence the character of a person (Guma 2001). For example, children are often given names that reflect the gratitude of the parents, such as Mpho (gift), Realeboha (we are thankful), and Rethabile (we are happy). Names that indicate positive traits are also common, such as Keneuoe (patience), Tlotliso (honor), and Keletso (advice), which was my Sesotho name.[5] If an infant is born following the death of a previous child, the child is often given a name that has more negative connotations, such as Ntja (dog) or some form of the name Tseliso (condolences). The underlying idea is to ensure the child's survival by indicating (falsely) that the child is not overly loved, thus deterring God or the ancestors from taking a beloved child away.[6]

The continued importance of children is a double-edged sword in rural Basotho communities. On one hand, the high value placed on children ensures that children are well cared for within the extended family network even in times of crisis. On the other hand, the priority placed on childbearing as a prerequisite to adulthood is true even for men and women living with HIV. In this way, the same values that bolster extended networks of kin and place an emphasis on caregiving also put children at risk of HIV infection and orphanhood.

## BLOOD, MILK, FOOD

The process of creating and maintaining relatedness is often connected to the mutable, fluid, and flexible creation of personhood through shared substance. The power of substances to shape and alter kin relations among Basotho has no exact correlate in Western societies. In North America, for example, blood contains the "true" imprint of biological relations, such as paternity. Other important substances, such as breastmilk and food, are seen in North America as healthful and symbolically important to familial relationships, but the power of a shared meal is in the companionship and the love and care put into the food, not in the food itself. In Lesotho, as in other places where kinship is not as firmly linked to biology, substances are both symbolically important and physically imbued with the power to shape and alter kin relations. In particular, shared blood, milk, and food provide means of creating kinship. As Carsten argues, the ways that substances are related to the formation and strengthening of kin ties are highly variable and bring together "a whole range of other themes including procreation, relations between kin, bodies, personhood, gender, and feeding" (2004, 132).

Surprisingly, blood was not emphasized by Basotho as an important shared substance, and when asked what makes someone close kin in general terms, people rarely mentioned blood. When I asked specifically about blood, several people shared with me the Sesotho expression "Mali a llelana" (Blood cries for blood). For older caregivers, blood symbolized a close kinship rather than a biological tie. When asked to list those with whom they shared blood, elderly caregivers often included their husbands and in-laws, many listed their closest relatives, and others focused on their *ngoaneso hantle* (real siblings). However, there was no uniform answer or overarching narrative about the exact role blood played in people's relationships, and when I asked one young mother who her blood relatives were, she replied, "*Ache*, I don't think it can happen."

Among Malays from Pulau Langkawi, Carsten (1995) noted the belief that one would not be able to receive blood from a sibling because the blood is too similar. In contrast, 'M'e Maliapeng, the widow living in her husband's village, told me that if she needed blood, she would have to go to her natal home to receive it. "If someone needs blood from someone," she explained, "I won't be given blood from one of these people, but they would prefer me to go to my home. They would prefer me to go to take my sibling's [blood] at my home. I will be given the blood from the one who has breastfed from the same mother." In this case, although she expresses a theory about shared blood, it is in the context of shared milk, which, as I show, is much more important as a unifying substance for people in Mokhotlong. Others noted that blood was important because it indicated someone who would "pity" you; that is, someone who would help you if you asked them. In the case of both older and younger caregivers, the substantiality of blood was not important, but rather, blood was alluded to as a symbolic representation of relatedness that indicated closeness and reciprocal responsibility. Again, the lived reality of kin relations surpassed any biologically determined markers of kinship. Like lineality, my interlocutors' ideas about blood were mutable reflections of their social reality.

Establishing and creating relatedness for Basotho is in part about the give and take of key substances—exchanges not possible with blood. In comparison to blood, caregivers I spoke with emphasized shared food and breastmilk as physically and symbolically transformative. Unlike blood, my interlocutors brought up the concept of shared breastmilk regularly—a key factor in creating a sympathetic relationship with their siblings and a marker for the closeness of a relationship, rather than evidence of it.

Basotho women do not routinely breastfeed any children but their own, so only biological siblings share breastmilk. Many women noted that they had "breastfed from the same mother" as a way of explaining how their relationship to their siblings was different from their relationship to their husbands' siblings. 'M'e Maphonolo mentioned breastfeeding as an indication of siblingship but recognized that this does not necessarily indicate the strength of a relationship in practice. She told me that to say someone is related to you means that you are siblings but does not mean that you are "children of the same stomach," who breastfed from the same mother. While she thought shared milk was important for sibling relationships, it was not all-powerful. "*Ache*," she told me, "it can happen that we are the children of the same mother but hate each other. And we don't go together at all. And someone who doesn't know us would not agree that we are children of the same mother." Ntate Kanelo and 'M'e Maliehi, the elderly grandparents of Matseli, had different opinions on this matter. 'M'e Maliehi thought that the closeness of siblings was perhaps related to breastfeeding. She told me, "*Ache*, it's because we have shared milk. And I don't know if milk makes love between people." In contrast, Ntate Kanelo thought that his close relationship with his siblings stemmed from their shared upbringing.

Breastfeeding is also viewed as an important practice that cements the mother-child bond. 'M'e Malefu, a village health worker, was caring for her deceased daughter's two teenaged girls. She had a very close relationship with her daughter before she died and cared for her in the late stages of AIDS. She felt that breastfeeding was an important way for mothers and children to bond "because it makes children to love their mothers. And the mothers, when they see their children, they feel pity for them. And also the children, when they see their mother, they have more love." I wanted to know if the breastmilk was the key bonding substance or if it was merely symbolic of a close relationship. To this end, I asked several caregivers about a scenario where a mother was unable to breastfeed one of her children, and in all cases, the caregivers responded that this did not change the relationship between the mother and child or between siblings. As 'M'e Malefu put it, "It's the love from the mother." In contrast, 'M'e Maliehi said it would cause her to feel "more pity"—that is, more compassion—for that sibling because she had lost her mother (she assumed that if a mother could not breastfeed, it was because the mother had died). This view emphasizes both the symbolic importance of breastfeeding and the flexibility of conceptions of shared substance as a means of physical transformation. In the context of HIV, where approximately one-third of mother-to-child transmission occurs through breastfeeding, the prevailing view of breast milk as wholly nutritive and unitive becomes even more complex, as I will address in chapter 3.

Food sharing has long been recognized in anthropology as a way of maintaining social connections, with more recent explorations demonstrating that food sharing is a way of expressing care and of making kin (Hutchinson 2000; Carsten 1995; Peluso 1996; Leinaweaver 2005). Food, like milk, is both nourishing and kin forming, but it also invokes the hospitality, courtesy, and morality of the domestic space. The potential for food to transform and shape relationships is more powerful than that of milk because it is not limited to mother-child and sibling bonds but instead encompasses bonds as diverse as those with extended kin, friends and neighbors, and ancestors. In Lesotho, high rates of food insecurity and malnutrition threaten these important kin-forming functions.

In Mokhotlong, people plant and harvest food with the help of family and neighbors in the land surrounding their homes. Ideally, rural Basotho families grow and harvest the majority of their own food from their fields and gardens. However, this has been increasingly difficult due to food insecurity caused by climate change, periodic droughts, soil erosion, and overgrazing (Himmelgreen et al. 2009; Leduka et al. 2015). Instead, most rural families are not food self-sufficient but rather combine their own harvests with food purchased from local shops and from food aid provided by various government programs and NGOs.

The preparation and distribution of food is a highly gendered domain in rural Lesotho. Men and women divvy up the tasks of ploughing, planting, and harvesting along gendered lines. While men slaughter animals for special feasts, women prepare all the food, including the meat. It is customary for Basotho women to serve men, who rarely if ever dish out their own food. Even at staff parties at MCS—where all leadership roles are held by women—the female employees, regardless of their positions in the organization, would form a line, dance in and out of the kitchen to speakers blasting *famo* or remixed American pop music, and serve food to the rest of the staff. Women are responsible for the nourishment of kin and the execution of hospitality, both in everyday life and during ritual occasions.

Food is a central and necessary component of ritual occasions. Events such as weddings and funerals center on a shared feast, which usually includes a slaughtered animal (often a sheep, although the type of animal depends on the wealth of the family and the number of expected guests). In addition, *papa* (maize meal), *moroho* (chopped, cooked greens), rice, other vegetables, and *joala* (home brew) are served. Before ARVs were widely available and AIDS-related deaths were more common, my friends in Mokhotlong attended a funeral most weekends, where they mourned the loss of a friend or family member, shared in a feast, and reconnected with those in their social networks. Although funeral costs were burdensome for most families, food sharing was considered an essential element of the occasion as well as a source of pride. Ritual occasions showcase the importance of food in cementing, reconnecting, and forming social bonds. Due to their social import and their symbolic richness, I will describe a few of them in detail here.

'M'e Masello cared for seven orphaned grandchildren, and during my fieldwork, I spent countless hours sitting with her. She was a raconteur of some exuberance, who would tell me elaborate stories, embellishing details and laughing loudly at her own jokes. She once described for me the funeral she held for her 12-year-old grandson, who had died unexpectedly of a brain aneurism. Throughout our conversation, she focused intently on the food she provided her guests. I have reproduced a portion of that conversation here, because 'M'e Masello humorously insisted on talking about the food at length, eschewing any attempts to steer the conversation elsewhere.

ELLEN: Were there many people at the funeral?

'M'E MASELLO: *Hele!* There were many people, as if he was an old person.[7] The meat ran out, yet they were only giving them one piece, one piece. It got finished.

ELLEN: Two whole sheep ran out?

'M'E MASELLO: Yes, two. But they did not finish the *joala* because there was much. They drank it until they were tired, and they came back on Sunday again. . . . And we had too much of sorghum porridge. . . . Yes, yes, 'M'e. It was good, very much. There were only white things. [The sheep] was fat. Mmm, hae, hae, hae!

ELLEN: So the boy came on Friday, and the funeral was on Saturday, and you made lots of food and ate two sheep. What else happened at the funeral?

'M'E MASELLO: I have forgotten that even beans were there. There were some people from my home who came with beans, *ache,* and there were many, because we still have them here at home. And they finished that pot of beans . . .

AUSI NTSOAKI: Yes, and what else happened at the funeral other than eating food?

'M'E MASELLO: I said pumpkin . . . and we slept.

AUSI NTSOAKI: Besides food, what else happened besides food?

'M'E MASELLO: Bread—and drinks. And Ntate Ntsele came with a big box and drinks and soup—the big one, which is mixed with other foods.

'M'e Masello, not known for her brevity, persisted until she was certain that she had listed everything that was served. The ability to hold such a bountiful feast for her grandson's funeral was not only a point of personal pride but, in the absence of wealth, an indication of her social connections and her strength as a hospitable head-of-household.

When I talked to people about the burden of funeral costs, most responded that although expensive, food was necessary in order to "accompany the person to the grave"—a common phrase used to describe the purpose of a funeral. The ritual requires much human labor—from digging the grave to carrying the coffin to numerous other kinds of logistical assistance—and all these people need to be fed. One chilly June day, 'M'e Masello and I sat outside on an old tarp in the sun, as we often did, pushing flavescent kernels of dried maize off a cob with our thumbs. 'M'e Masello was lamenting the financial burden of a recent funeral (not her grandson's described earlier), when I naively suggested that perhaps such elaborate funerals were not necessary. She reproached me sharply, "Even if you are too poor to provide meat," she told me, "you should provide something." Yet many—like 'M'e Masello, whose own health was poor and who was caring for seven orphaned grandchildren in one small rondavel—made immense sacrifices to provide a feast, despite their poverty. I never attended or heard of a funeral that did not have meat, regardless of the poverty of the family.

While food sharing has the power to draw friends and relatives closer, it can also be used to create distance between kin. The absence of food sharing or the refusal to share food is highly destructive to relationships. 'M'e Matshepo, a young woman who was having problems with her husband, described a major conflict when he refused to eat food that she had served him:

> There was a funeral for the child of my sister-in-law, and when I was going to give [my husband] food, because the food was finished, he refused to take it. And I went back crying because I was very angry. And I told my brother because he was there at the funeral. And my mother-in-law was very angry. His mother said she doesn't know what to do because he's old, and she can't beat him. I'm always telling her that the life I'm living is so difficult. And sometimes he doesn't buy me some shoes, and sometimes I go where he is working and report all the things that he is doing, and there are many things that make me angry. I can talk for a long time.

'M'e Matshepo's husband refusing food was seen, even by his own mother, as an extremely disrespectful action to take against his wife and especially humiliating in a public setting such as a funeral. 'M'e Matshepo also told me on numerous occasions that her husband had failed to bring food money for her and her two children, and she was required to ask his family for help. Through these actions, 'M'e Matshepo's husband was severing important ties that are made and maintained in part by shared food. His refusal to eat what she had served him was a way of opting out of a caring exchange. She viewed it as equally egregious as not providing money to feed his children. Because of the importance of food sharing and the wife's role as the cook and server of food, his refusal went beyond a mere marital dispute to the core of their relationship and the relationship between the two families. It indicated significant strife between the couple, who later separated.

The transformative power of food is not limited to relations between living persons but is carried into people's relationships with ancestors. Food is the primary substance used to connect the living with the dead. Honoring ancestors through food offerings, similar to the importance of accompanying the deceased to the grave, is not only about respect and honor but about maintaining ideals of lineality. Basotho remember their ancestors, especially during the harvest season, when food is in abundance, by cooking for them and brewing *joala* (which, when brewed for the purpose of honoring ancestors, is called *mohlaba*).[8] 'M'e Marefiloe, the great-grandmother of Nkhabu, described this offering: "When I'm brewing *mohlaba*, when I pour the water in the drum, I will talk and say—I will call [my ancestors] by their clans; I will start with my family and the family where I'm married, my husband and his children who have died, and say, 'Here are the foods; I'm making them for you.'" Many of my interlocutors, particularly the younger ones, said that they no longer believed in ancestors but instead believed in God. However, many self-identified Christian elderly caregivers saw these two belief systems as compatible. 'M'e Maliehi, the grandmother of Matseli, who went to the Catholic church regularly and was part of a women's group and choir there, still cooked for her ancestors, combining her beliefs in God and what many call "Sesotho culture" in a creative way. She told me,

> Sometimes, when I have cooked the food, and I call my friends and neighbors, and I will say, "I have called you here to all be happy. And I have cooked also for the grandfathers and grandmothers, and we should also be happy with them. And those who are not there." After we have cooked the food, we take one plate, and we put everything, everything, everything that we have cooked on it, and we put them there outside. And we pray for them. And we say, "We have cooked for the dead people and the living people." And they will be eaten by old people. Not [just] anyone.[9]

When 'M'e Maliehi referred to "grandfathers and grandmothers," the kinship networks invoked by this terminology include ancestors. She believed that mentioning the ancestors' names was important when receiving help from God. In this way, she conceived of her ancestors much like Catholic saints who could help intercede with God on her behalf, and food played an essential role in reaching them.

The moral dimension of food sharing and its potential to uphold or dissolve social and familial relationships intersect with growing food insecurity and HIV in Lesotho. As Himmelgreen and his colleagues (2009) argue, HIV and food insecurity are syndemic: they intersect in complex overlapping ways with gender inequality, transactional sex, malnutrition, and immune function. Other studies show that food insecurity is linked to poor ARV adherence, since exacerbated hunger is a side effect of the medications. Food insecurity also impacts the nutrition of breastfeeding infants and young children cared for by people living with HIV (Young et al. 2014). While I explore the effects of food insecurity and child malnutrition in greater ethnographic detail in chapter 3, the connections between the moral and social dimensions of food sharing are intimately linked to poverty and growing food insecurity.

## CARING INSTITUTIONS: MARRIAGE, NATAL KIN, AND AFFINAL KIN

The act of raising and caring for children is not merely about the physical exchange of substances or the change in social position that comes with parenthood. It is a key social exchange that fosters and shapes the emotional ties between people. Young women in particular have strong emotional attachments to their natal kin as compared to their affinal kin (i.e., in-laws, or relatives through marriage). Patrilineal societies, including the Basotho, prefer patrilocal residence patterns, where a newly married couple sets up their home in the husband's village, near his parents. In contemporary Lesotho, couples might live in town for work, move to the city, or reside with the wife's kin, for social and economic reasons. Yet even when these idealized residence patterns are adhered to, closeness among natal kin does not end with marriage or relocation but continues into adulthood even as young people get married, move, have children, and form new ties with extended networks of kin. Basotho maintain the relationships with and social obligations to those who have raised them and cared for them. In the anthropological literature on the cultural construction of emotion, scholars of southern Africa have noted that love is not merely a feeling but an act of doing (Klaits 2010; Durham and Klaits 2002; Alverson 1978). In large part because of the social consequences of HIV/AIDS, the social geography of relationships between people is gradually shifting, with less emphasis on affinal ties, increased emphasis on care, and the emergence of the house as a crossroads where raising and caring present the most stable form of social and emotional investment.

Basotho are affectionate with their children, talk about love between married partners, and emphasize the strong love that exists between grandparents and grandchildren. However real these feelings are, affection and love are also culturally produced. Emotions are, in part, socially constructed narratives that reflect caring relationships (Manderson and Block 2016). My interlocutors generally discussed their relationships with their natal kin in terms of love, affection, and pity, while describing their relationships with their affinal kin more in terms of duty. These affective dynamics illuminate why, in times of distress, women increasingly turn first toward their natal rather than their affinal kin. Most women initially said there was no difference between their natal and affinal families, but once we started discussing the matter, they revealed attitudes about their in-laws characterized largely by a sense of reciprocal responsibility, which was amplified if bridewealth had been paid. The nature of these relationships was closely linked to the fact that women often live and work in their husbands' villages, houses, and fields. Because of proximity and mutual responsibility, in-laws are the people to whom women usually turn when they need something material (such as maize meal, soap, or money for transportation), but they turn toward their natal kin for more intensive and intimate caregiving needs. People verbalized this by using terms like *love* or *pity* when describing their natal kin; these feelings are more conducive to the kind of long-term care that an orphan or sick adult would require. In general, the relationship between a woman and her natal kin—parents, siblings, and grandparents—was described as loving and supportive. When marriages fall apart or when a husband dies, young women often turn to their parents or grandparents for assistance because they feel that they will be more sympathetic. This is especially true in the context of weakened marriage bonds and the shortened life span of young adults in Lesotho.

Older married women were more firmly established in their married homes and therefore, over time, developed deeper emotional and material attachments to their affinal kin. Even when the husband was deceased or the husband and wife were estranged, an older woman was more likely than a young one to remain at her married home. 'M'e Matau is a woman in her 60s for whom these sentiments toward kin were evident. When I asked her about the differences between her natal and affinal kin, she said, "*Ache*, there is no difference, but they have the difference of cows [bridewealth]." Then, however, she elaborated that her siblings were "on top" of her husband's siblings. Like many Basotho, she used the word *pity* (*mohau*) to mean some combination of love, empathy, and charity. She said her siblings (as opposed to her siblings-in-law) felt a deeper "pity" for each other: "It's because they are the children that I have grown up with. . . . They feel pity for each other because one will say, 'This is my sibling,' because they have grown up together." Yet if she needed assistance with food or money, she would ask her husband's family first because, as she put it, "It's where I live," indicating the mutual responsibility that comes with marriage, particularly when bridewealth has been paid.

Thapo's grandmother, 'M'e Masekha, did not express a difference in her feelings toward her natal and affinal kin but regarded her married home as the one where she had many responsibilities. When I asked her about this difference, she said, "I do everything here alone." I then asked her if she ever went to her own brothers and sisters for help. "Yes," she told me, "if I need something, I go, and they help me. I don't like to go often [to ask for help]. I want them to be happy when I go." In this way, 'M'e Masekha indicated that she preferred not to ask for assistance from her natal kin so that her visits could remain primarily social. Being long married and well established at the village of her affines allowed her this advantage. Younger and recently married caregivers might not be able to navigate this as easily.

'M'e Maphonolo is a young woman, separated from her husband, who lives with her three children and two of her much younger brothers (for whom she had cared since their parents died several years prior). Her youngest daughter, Lintle, an MCS client, was conceived after 'M'e Maphonolo and her husband separated, although he is listed as the father on MCS's intake form. 'M'e Maphonolo suggested that the distinction between one's own siblings and one's husband's siblings was relevant only if there was enmity: "I can say these ones are the ones where I'm married, and these ones, where I'm born," she told me. "I can say that if I don't love them." She also said that when she was married, she had more responsibilities to her in-laws because "she had gone there by cow," meaning bridewealth was paid. In her case, the estrangement and separation from her husband created tension with the rest of her in-laws, so she moved back to her natal home after her divorce.

'M'e Nthabiseng also explained that tension with affinal kin, particularly between a woman and her mother-in-law, was common. This tension, combined with the decline in customs like bridewealth payment—which helped maintain alliances between families—had resulted in a shift toward matrilocal patterns of orphan care. Several caregivers also cited tension with a mother-in-law as a primary reason women might look to their natal families for support. One morning, Ausi Ntsoaki and I drove my motorbike to the far end of town to deliver supplies to Tebello, an orphaned child who had lived in the MCS safe home and was now an outreach client. He lived with his paternal uncle and was primarily cared for by the uncle's young wife, 18-year-old 'M'e Masenate. She and her neighbor, 'M'e Matsiu, also married and in her late teens, were sitting in her small row house while Tebello played on the linoleum floor, dressed in a new burgundy sweat suit that MCS had given him. After delivering the supplies, we sat on the bed and chatted for a while. Although both women were young and newly married, 'M'e Masenate had a particularly strained relationship with her mother-in-law. When I asked her why this was the case, she mused, "I don't know. Sometimes we might see that the mother-in-law is acting silly toward the daughter-in-law or the daughter-in-law is silly to the mother-in-law," referring to tensions over housework, child care, and claims on the husband's time, as well as general attitudes toward each other. Her friend, 'M'e Matsiu, piped in, "I have seen that when the daughter-in-law is being silly to the mother-in-law, they will always fight. And if there is a girl in that family, the girl will be silly, and the mothers always listen to their daughters. If the daughter-in-law is good, they don't care." Even though both of these women acknowledged that a daughter-in-law's behavior could at least partly contribute to the tension, they indicated that a mother-in-law might dislike her daughter-in-law whether or not she was causing any problems. These tensions tend to recede as women establish themselves more firmly in their married homes with the birth of children and as the older generation of in-laws age and pass away.

In contrast to her friend, 'M'e Matsiu had a strong relationship with her affinal kin, and her opinions were colored by her own experiences. She was orphaned as a teenager and indicated that she felt more supported by her in-laws than by older relatives on her side of the family. Despite being helped by her in-laws, she still admitted stronger feelings of love for her own siblings. She laughed, "My siblings are troublesome, but I love them more than my husband's siblings. I love them more than those ones. Maybe it's because we have grown up together." These strong feelings of love, in contrast with the tensions inherent in relationships with affinal kin, help explain the shift toward matrilocal care during difficult times. Because HIV/AIDS has had the greatest impact on young married people, who are more likely to have young children, women often turn toward their natal kin to help care for them during their illness and to look after their children if they do not recover.

There is general agreement among both young and old people in Mokhotlong that marriage is no longer taken as seriously as it was in the past but that divorce (*lifolose*) is a foreign concept that does not fit with Sesotho cultural ideals (Ntimo-Makara 2009). 'M'e Maphonolo's brief marriage to her husband demonstrates some of the complex ways that the bonds of marriage have weakened because of the changing economic and cultural landscape. 'M'e Maphonolo is the woman introduced previously who was caring for her three children and two much younger brothers. In her mid-20s, she moved back to her natal village when her marriage ended. Unlike most young couples in Lesotho today who marry for love, 'M'e Maphonolo was "stolen" by her husband. In this practice of *chobeliso* (loosely translated as "abduction"), a man, helped by friends or relatives, goes into a girl's home or waits for her along a path he knows she will be traveling, then physically carries her back to his village and consummates the marriage.

'M'e Maphonolo said that she could have left her marriage right away if she wanted to, but she decided to stay, and she was, she told me, happy for a while. After a short time, however, her husband left for work in South Africa, and she returned to her natal village. She said, "What is the use of being there when there is no one taking care of me? And there were no cows [meaning bridewealth]. And I came back." Despite this ominous beginning and although she did not return to live in his village, 'M'e Maphonolo remained married to her husband and had two children. But his frequent and lengthy absences in South Africa put a strain on their marriage, which was not strongly established.

The marriage started to turn when her family began asking for bridewealth. She explained, "It happened like this. My parents needed cows from his father. And his father said he would bring his son to come back home. And his son told him that he will not come back home at all. He's going to stay in Natal [South Africa]. And his father told me that 'He has another wife, your husband.' And I told myself that I'm going back home." In 'M'e Maphonolo's case, a hasty non-consensual marriage, separation due to migrant labor, the absence of bride-wealth, and her husband's infidelity all created insurmountable obstacles to the success of the union. When I asked her if she wanted to get married again, she replied, "I have had it, and it's enough." She views the institution of marriage as fundamentally different from when her parents and grandparents were young:

> *Ache!* We [young people] are just playing. Or it's because I was married while still young. Or I was married without a good mind. Without a good mind. I don't know. I don't know what happened because I didn't like it. To be married, I didn't like it. . . . Old people really had a good marriage, *kannete* [I swear]. Because they are still saying that, even when looking at them, you can see that. They were living very well. But, no, ah ah, *kannete*, we are not. . . . Love, *ngoaneso* [my dear], is gone now. It is not there at all, at all, at all, love. It is gone. Gone, gone, gone, gone.

'M'e Maphonolo's sentiments about marriage were echoed by many other women, both young and old. A common phrase mentioned by both genera-tions was that "there is no more love" and that in the past, people were more patient (*keneuoe*) in their marriages, which in many cases meant the tolerance of infidelity and long stretches of separation. Although many younger caregivers remember their parents and grandparents as being happier in their marriages, the older women admitted to conflict. 'M'e Marefiloe, who was 78, reflected the general sentiment of older women: "Old people were always happy at their mar-riage. And even when it was difficult, they were patient. But these ones are not patient. . . . *Ache, ngoanaka* [my dear], nowadays, there is no marriage." While Tsepi's grandmother, 'M'e Matau, remembered being happy in her marriage, she also said that she sometimes fought with her husband and occasionally threat-ened to leave him: "Sometimes I left him and went to my home. I would go back to my home, and he would come to collect me. I was going to leave him. But we had children, and we stopped fighting." Marriage, like other markers of kinship, is a process. Once their marriage was solidified by the birth of children, the con-flict between them ceased to be a cause for separation.

Many older women said their own families contributed to their marital sta-bility. When fighting with their husbands, women recalled returning to their natal families until the conflict subsided. The couple's parents would then work to bring the spouses back together. For example, 'M'e Maliehi, Matseli's grandmother, explained that her relatives encouraged her to stay in her marriage. She told me, "The mother or the grandmother would just say, 'You should be patient, my daughter.' And they said, 'You must do good things for your husband to be happy. You must be patient.'"

Of course, not all elderly people had successful marriages. Ntate Kapo was deserted by his wife when his children were still very young. He raised his children by himself and later raised his deceased daughter's two sons, one of whom was HIV positive. Although they never divorced, Ntate Kapo's wife started a new family in the lowlands of Lesotho, and he had not seen her for over 20 years. 'M'e Malefu—an elderly village health worker and caregiver for two teenaged orphans—was also separated from her husband. She lived in his family's village, where she had been for many years, and he occasionally came to visit, but he stayed elsewhere, and they no longer shared resources. When I asked 'M'e Malefu in 2009 if she wanted him to come back, she revealed that she was worried about contracting HIV from him: "It's better if he is living there. I don't want him to come back because he will bring some diseases to me."

Because 'M'e Malefu was a village health worker, she viewed her husband's absence as beneficial not only financially but also for her health. When I returned to visit her in 2015, she invited me to her village for a lunch of *papa*, *moroho*, and peach chutney. As we sipped on warm Coke and waited for the *papa* to cook, she told me that her husband had returned to her the previous year, sick and in need of care. She did not refuse him and nursed him for a year before he died. Unlike many of the younger women I spoke with, 'M'e Malefu was dedicated both to her marriage and to the institution of marriage, even though she and her husband did not always cohabitate.

Many of the younger women I knew in Mokhotlong were divorced, separated, or never married. In contrast, only two of the elderly caregivers I spent the most time with were separated, although many were widowed. These trends are influenced by the increased potential for women to earn money for their households and the increased educational opportunities for women in Lesotho, which lead to a delayed average age at first marriage and overall lower marriage rates (Lesotho Ministry of Health 2016). Researchers have shown that women's education delays the age at first marriage, and Lesotho has had high rates of girls in school for decades (Timaeus and Graham 1989). Those who saw education as a positive factor for couples viewed it as a general good and therefore extrapolated that it would be beneficial to marriage. 'M'e Mamohato viewed education as taking the strain off a marriage by giving couples some independence: "If one is a nurse and one is a teacher and we all go for work, I just think it's better. We cannot easily be fighting because we are not always together. You would just be together for a short time." Those who saw it as a drawback pointed to the temptation of having other partners outside of marriage, especially when spouses were differently educated. What is certain is that education decreases the dependence of women on men for their livelihood. As 'M'e Maliehi stated, "If the husband is doing things the wife doesn't want, the wife will just say, 'I don't care. I'm going because I'm educated.'"

'M'e Nthabiseng thought that increased access to legal representation—and women's reluctance to stay in abusive relationships—led to divorce. Like many of my interlocutors, 'M'e Nthabiseng, who raised her son without the help of his father, did not see divorce as problematic but saw it as something that enabled women to escape unhappy and potentially unsafe relationships. While divorce rates have been more stable than marriage rates in Lesotho, people's experience with marital dissolution has increased, and many point to the changing relations between men and women as a probable cause.

Political-economic circumstances such as high rates of migrant labor, apartheid, and the AIDS pandemic have all contributed to this changing landscape of marriage and affinal kin ties (Murray 1981; Coplan 1987; Romero-Daza and Himmelgreen 1998; Modo 2001), fundamentally altering the role of marriage in creating and maintaining social ties. The expanded social relations that one accrues as one ages are highly subject to changing social geography. Social demographics such as marriage, the birth of children, and the exchange of bridewealth used to be good markers along the processual road to adulthood. This is no longer the case. Although the emerging instability of these social markers has created increased vulnerability, it has also revealed adaptability in finding new ways to establish and maintain important relationships, including the provision of care for orphans.

## BRIDEWEALTH REVISITED

One aspect of the institution of marriage that requires close investigation is the exchange of bridewealth, which, until recently, was extremely common among Basotho (Turkon 2003). My interlocutors were of mixed opinion when it came to the role that bridewealth played in strengthening marriage bonds. Like other cultural ideals, of course, bridewealth payments have never been uniform or consistent. However, decreased marriage rates, the reduced importance of formal marital unions, and the waning migrant labor market have made bridewealth payments less common and more prohibitive for young people and therefore less potent as a cultural ideal. The decline in bridewealth in some ways may cause instability, but it also creates opportunities for new patterns of relatedness in a way that privileges care over lineality.

Traditionally, bridewealth (*likhomo*—Sesotho for "cows") was ideally paid from the man's family to the woman's family. As Basotho marriage is a process more than an event, there would typically be an initial payment at the time of the marriage, with more cows arriving over time. In some cases, with very wealthy families, most or all of the cows would be paid at the time of marriage—a noteworthy accomplishment for both families. A couple may move in together without a ceremony, but the exchange of even one cow signals the beginning of the marriage. Couples may have a Sesotho ceremony in their village, a church ceremony (often called a "white wedding"), or some combination of the two. Although many marriages are registered with the government, they are socially and legally recognized even when not notarized by the state. Usually, *likhomo* payment is established with reference to a certain number of cows agreed upon by the families of the couple prior to the union, but a payment of cash or equivalent goods is a viable substitute. Even when the payment is made in cash or goods, it is counted in cows and so is called by the Sesotho name *likhomo*. For many older women, the number of cows their in-laws provided and the speed with which they were delivered were points of pride.

Both young and old Basotho agree that the practice of *likhomo* has changed. In general, people pay fewer cows, if any, and these are often promised but not paid in full. Ntate Kapo's elderly and blind mother, 'M'e Matlotliso, usually sat outside her rondavel all day, enjoying the sun and talking to passersby. Ausi Ntsoaki and I approached her one day, looking for Ntate Kapo, who had gone to work in the fields. She said that she would like to talk to us, so we waited while she painstakingly followed a wire that Ntate Kapo had put between her rondavel and the outhouse so she could use the toilet when he was gone. 'M'e Matlotliso was in her late 70s, and she was confused by the changes that had taken place in Lesotho during her lifetime. When I asked her about HIV, she claimed that she knew very little, even though she lived next door to her grandson, who was on ARVs. However, when I asked her about changes in marriage and *likhomo*, she had a strong opinion:

> *Ache*, nowadays, they don't pay *likhomo*. They just take the girls. If they pay one, *kannete*, they have paid *likhomo*. Or if they have paid two or three, you must know that they have paid a lot, oh ho! [*laughs*] And sometimes they take the girl for some years, not paying anything. . . . And the girls nowadays are just married without paying *likhomo*. If they can take care of my children and be good to my children . . . ah ah, no problem. I have seen it happening like that. . . . There is a difference in [marriage] nowadays because they don't pay anything for the children. At least, in our age, there was something paid. And they gave it to our parents, because they were the ones caring for us.

'M'e Matlotliso, it became clear, saw a direct link between *likhomo* payment and care. It not only solidified the economic responsibility of families but recognized the care and support required by children.

Some caregivers made a direct connection between the decrease in *likhomo* payments and the increased instability of marriage. 'M'e Mamohato was a young woman who still lived in her husband's village with her three children, although he was deceased and although she did not get along with her mother-in-law, because she enjoyed the independence of running her own household. However, she saw the lack of bridewealth exchange as contributing to her independence. When I asked 'M'e Mamohato if she thought old people were happier in their marriages, she said, "Even if they were not happy, the fact that *likhomo* was paid . . . it's not like now. I can now go at my home because there was nothing paid. I could just take my children and go, but the fact that I have my own house, I won't go anywhere. And it's easy for me because no one will say, 'Where are you going with these children?'" Yet when I asked her why there was more divorce, she told me, "Nowadays, because there is no *likhomo*. If *likhomo* is paid, the parents can stand between to make those people stay together. And they will say, 'My cows have gone out, so go back to your marriage.' But nowadays, they just get divorced, and no one stands between them. Because there is no *likhomo*." Like many of my interlocutors, 'M'e Mamohato found herself in the occasionally uneasy liminal space of a culture shift: lamenting the loss of traditional forms of social stability while enjoying the freedom of increased independence—an especially potent experience for a Mosotho woman.

Not all women blamed increasing marital instability on the decrease of *likhomo*. Many gave examples of those who stayed in their marriages even when *likhomo* was not paid or those who left when it had been paid. When I asked 'M'e Mapoloko, 77, if she thought a decrease in *likhomo* payment was a factor in the changing state of marriage, she said, "Is it so? I don't know because I have seen with some people that *likhomo* are not paid, but they are still living with their husbands. But some, they just marry one today, and tomorrow, they marry another one, just like that. Because they are lazy, they did not work for *likhomo*." For 18-year-old 'M'e Masenate, no *likhomo* had been paid at the time of her marriage because her husband did not make enough money to cover their monthly expenses in addition to *likhomo*. Recently, she and her husband had been fighting, and she informed me that she was considering leaving him. I asked if she thought a woman would be less likely to leave if *likhomo* had been paid. "Ah ah," she said. "*Kannete* [I swear], if you feel like going, you must go."

Despite these differences of opinion, *likhomo* payments have both a historical and a contemporary importance in creating bonds between families. In reality, it is unlikely that 'M'e Masenate would be as free to leave her husband if *likhomo* had been paid, due to cultural pressures and the intervention of her family.[10] Extended families are more invested in the success of marriages where *likhomo* have been paid, in part because the process of untangling the marriage and bridewealth is complicated (e.g., cows received from a daughter's marriage may have already left the family to pay bridewealth for a son's marriage). Parents were more frequently involved in bringing a quarrelling couple back together when *likhomo* was paid. In some ways, the breakdown of marriage customs has made families unstable by creating less support within the immediate family—however, a decrease in *likhomo* payments in particular has made it possible for maternal families to care for orphaned children without violating the idealized rules of patrilineality (a topic to which I return in chapter 4). It has also given young women (and men) greater autonomy in deciding the fate of their marriages. In place of more firmly established marriages and *likhomo* payments, the house has become an increasingly stable and binding milieu for Basotho, a place where other key aspects of relatedness, such as lineality and substance, emerge and intersect. It is the dominant social institution of the house to which I now turn.

## HOUSES AND HOUSE LIFE

Houses and households are important in shaping relatedness based on the commonality of lived experience. Even as other changes in society are taking place, the house remains paramount as a space that frames human actions and transforms people's relationships—whether through physical proximity or acts of caregiving or as a place of shared substance. The house is a reflection of the social order; the physical structure, the members within it, the objects that fill cabinets and lie beneath beds—all of these comment on the tensions of the outside world. The house that shelters during wartime is not the house that shelters during periods of abundance; the house during the era of migrant labor is not the house of the AIDS pandemic. It is always a crossroads, a site of human movement, where fostering, marriage, and migration reorganize its inhabitants. In this way, the house is a nurturing space, weaving physical connections and emotional bonds into a tighter fabric. Most significantly, the house is where the labor of care takes place—those large and small acts that range from periods of intense care during illness to moments of absolute mundanity: wiping a child's nose, changing a diaper, or soothing a crying baby. Yet the house is not merely a passive site in the process of caring; it is a necessary strategic space where people actively shape kinship networks through intentional acts of care and neglect. While many ethnographic examples defy an explanation of the household as a coresidence (Yanagisako 1979), the demographic pressure of AIDS has reasserted the primacy of the house as the locus of caregiving labor and the place where kin relations are made and unmade.

The HIV epidemic has encoded itself into the rural landscape in unexpected ways. One might expect the AIDS house to be an abandoned space of disease, death, and collapse—and sometimes this is the case. However, through my observations of everyday practice in many Basotho houses, I witnessed the house as a durable space, one that can withstand the pressure of AIDS in order to facilitate care. The house has become a compressed space—quite literally—as houses are crowded with orphaned children and cluttered with the signs of care-giving, funerals, the materials that accompany household migration, and AIDS. The house serves as a clinic, a hospice, a halfway house, and a foster home. And while it has always performed these functions to an extent, AIDS has compressed the house's different caregiving roles in a way that is unprecedented in frequency and intensity. AIDS-related changes on the house can only be understood as exceptional in the context of such a widespread disturbance. While the house is only one component of caregiving, acting both as a shelter and a space where many acts of care take place, its role as a densely important social space has intensified.

The house's transformation under the pressure of HIV/AIDS has been rapid and intense. As described earlier, the HIV prevalence rate in Lesotho rose from nearly zero to 23 percent in less than a decade (UNAIDS 2010). This was expo-nentially faster than other external household pressures in Lesotho, most nota-bly migrant labor and its fluctuations over more than a century (Kimble 1982; Murray 1981). Of course, not all of the increased pressure from AIDS is felt in the house. AIDS's impact reverberates through lineages and other social institu-tions, including villages, clinics, schools, orphanages, and churches. But AIDS is intertwined with the physical space of the house in ways not seen beyond it. The ability for the house to withstand this extra pressure and respond to the care-giving needs of kin shows the resilience of the house as a social institution and its importance in maintaining networks of kin, keeping family members—albeit different ones—together. The reorganization of families around household units also reveals how, under duress, care becomes a primary organizing principle of social life. In taking on this extra pressure, the house is caring not only for kin—but for kinship itself.

In providing for children, caregivers create strong social bonds that are shaped and constrained by the spaces where care takes place. The "inhabited space"—namely, the house—is where children learn the embodiment of prac-tice (Bourdieu 1977, 89). I employ a "dwelling" perspective of the house (Hei-degger 1971), as opposed to merely a "building" perspective,[11] where "the forms people build . . . only arise within the current of their life activities" (Ingold 2000, 154). Outside the house, the nature and quality of care for children is far more difficult to discern. While it may be possible to infer signs of neglect based on a child's appearance, these signs are often confounded by poverty. It is inside the home where care—and neglect, fracturing, and anomie—is most readily experienced and observed.

Care is shaped by the physical structure of the home because of the ways in which space allows and constrains activities that take place within it (Birdwell-Pheasant and Lawrence-Zúñiga 1999). The caregiving that takes place in urban homes is in many ways similar to care in rural villages, yet it differs in a few key aspects. First, proximity to the district hospital and the road makes the transportation of a sick family member easier. Also, caregivers are more likely to be employed if they live in town, due to greater opportunities for wage labor. Children living in urban homes are thus more likely to be cared for by a neighbor during the day or to attend a home daycare or preschool, although in some cases, adults may live and work in town while some or all of their children remain with relatives in the village. Yet many children live with grandparents in town, and their daily care is attended to in many of the same ways as in rural villages; this is particularly so for young children, whose needs are prolonged and numerous.

Houses in the town of Mokhotlong and other urban and peri-urban areas are predominantly square structures made of cement, cinder blocks, and corrugated tin roofing or tiles. While village houses are typically owned by the families living in them, urban and peri-urban houses are often rented. Houses in town are more likely to include amenities such as small propane heating units, electricity, water, and gas burners or ovens due to increased incomes through employment and better infrastructure. Urban housing may have small vegetable gardens, but field space on the outskirts of town is limited. The majority of Basotho living in town also have rural houses and fields that belong to them or their families, which are occupied by kin and that they often visit during the harvest, returning home with their allotment of maize, wheat, or sorghum. While there are an increasing number of multichambered cinder-block dwellings across Lesotho's rural highlands—due to a desire for more space and aspirations of "modernity" (Ferguson 2006)—rondavels are still the dominant "house" in rural villages, which lack electricity, plumbing, and infrastructure.

Rural households typically consist of two or more houses, a garden for leafy greens and root vegetables, and nearby fields growing staple crops like maize and wheat (figure 1.4). These households are situated in villages with as few as 10 units to more than 100. While households within villages may be quite close together, they are demarcated in ways that create a yard-like space around each house, with structural additions that delineate the space, such as poles and laundry lines, planted bushes, low rock walls, empty Coke-bottle barriers, and rocky keyhole-shaped garden beds. These exterior structures increase the space controlled by the family and provide an outdoor area for socializing and shared housework such as laundry, crop preparation, and cooking. These elements of the landscape are considered part of a household's inheritance.

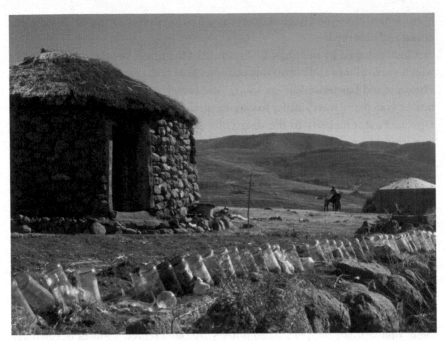

FIGURE 1.4. Exterior of rondavel, Mokhotlong, 2009

The outer walls of rondavels are made of large stones, the insides plastered with a thick impasto of insulating mud and dung; overhead, bundles of wheat or grass are carefully layered atop conical roofbeams. The interiors of rondavels in rural communities are relatively standard (figure 1.5). They usually consist of a small cooking hearth, which is dug approximately six inches into the floor. A collection of pots, storage containers, plates, and cups are usually neatly stacked along one wall, and this area is often decorated with plastic tablecloths, cutouts from newspapers, colorful flyers or posters, or calendars given away at clinics and shops. Men typically build houses, although women participate in collecting materials. While household members often build their houses with the help of kin and neighbors, new houses are increasingly built by hired local experts, skilled in the difficult task of securing suitable walls and thatching for the rain, wind, and snow. Rondavels are praised for their ability to retain heat in the winter and remain cool in the summer, which aids in maintaining health and providing care. The materials needed to build and repair them are collected in the surrounding areas, so rural Basotho prefer them to cement houses.

The house—whether rural or urban—is a moralized space of respect and honor, replete with social courtesies (Beidelman 1972; Feeley-Harnik 1980) best viewed from within the house. People's homes are almost always immaculately clean, a necessity in such crowded living spaces. Because my visits were

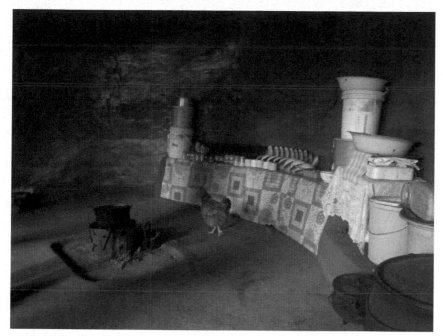

FIGURE 1.5. Inside of rondavel, Mokhotlong, 2009

often unexpected, I was frequently asked to wait outside so that my host could sweep or put away dishes from the previous meal. Almost without exception, hosts collected chairs or benches from neighbors if they did not have their own—a courtesy given to all visitors from outside the village. I was occasionally offered prepared food or given a plastic bag filled with freshly picked beans or spinach to take home. One maternal grandfather, Ntate Kapo, with whom I met frequently, was proud of his home and its spartan furnishings but lamented the condition of one of his tables. He told me, "The legs [of my table] are looking like the legs of an elephant. And they get broken. I want to have a carpet and chairs and a table so that the visitors like you can sit on them, and you are now just sitting on a bench. The important people like you."

Ntate Kapo's concerns attest to the importance of the house as a social space where hospitality is given. His description of an abandoned home emphasizes the sheltering and caring quality of houses: "I have seen that if you go and live somewhere else, your home will be turned to shambles, and the rats will live in it. . . . That's why I have been living here. . . . And when it has fallen down, I will have nowhere to live." For Ntate Kapo and others, the home is a place where one is rooted and where one must dwell in order to maintain those roots. Although interhousehold movement is common, the maintenance of the house by resident members helps orient both the inhabitants and the migrants who call it home.

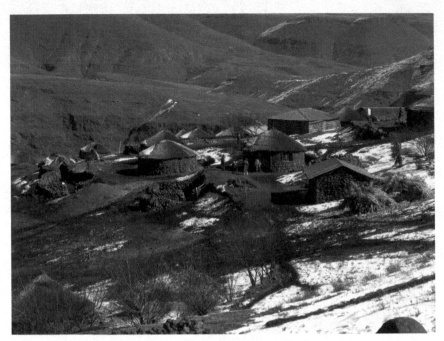

FIGURE 1.6. Rural village one week after a snowstorm, Mokhotlong, 2007

Houses also hold particular significance for the health and well-being of their inhabitants. This is evident both in the regular maintenance and care of houses and the concern over their collapse. 'M'e Mamolupe was caring for her brother-in-law's three children, who relocated from their father's house after he died. She pointed across the road, down the hill toward the houses where the children were born, indicating the new outhouse that she had just installed. She told me that she had one of her young, unmarried cousins living in those houses so that they would not fall apart while the children were too young to live there by themselves. 'M'e Mamolupe explained, "I didn't want their family to be deserted. I don't like that family to be dead. This 'M'e who is sitting there is the one; I put her there to live, to protect those houses. Which means I am look-ing out for these children who are growing up." Here 'M'e Mamolupe equates the houses with family and cares for them so that the orphans will inherit property, reinforcing the inseparability of financial and familial value. Like its inhabitants, the house is both a giver and receiver of care and is an increasingly important space in the context of AIDS.

One of the most tangible ways of tracing household change is through memory and material possessions, as the house is "a fascinating repository of culture and meaning" (Bahloul 1996, 2). In Lesotho, houses stand as historical (social) witnesses to the marked contrast between former (perceived) financial and physical well-being and health and current conditions of impoverishment and ill health. The legacy of migrant labor is revealed by a closer look at the symbolically significant artifacts of a more affluent time—items that power-fully evoke memories (Miller 2001; Olsen 2010). As Morton (2007) suggests, it is insufficient to think of the house as merely a vessel for memory, but rather, it must be regarded as active in the process of remembering through building and rebuilding. In Mokhotlong, the husbands of most elderly caregivers worked in the gold mines, and the remnants of this prosperous time are reflected within their houses. Extra items such as bookshelves, cupboards, broken clocks, draw-ers, wooden trunks, teacups and saucers, and tables reflect a period of greater influx of cash into the local economy.

Many elderly caregivers remembered migrant labor as a time of relative pros-perity when they had easy access to cash, often forgetting the struggle of separa-tion that characterized that time (Edkins et al. 1990; Epprecht 1993; Gordon 1994; Murray 1981). While treasured, their now-defunct and even cumber-some possessions—which take up precious space in small living quarters—are reminders of that time. Measurement tools used to assess household wealth in developing countries routinely use such durable goods as wealth indicators (Grosh and Glewwe 1995). Such an assessment in rural Mokhotlong would be misleading concerning a family's current wealth and access to cash, which are fundamentally tied to their ability to perform caregiving tasks. In many cases, elderly widows, whose homes are filled with such treasures, have very little income beyond their limited old-age pensions, and they often struggle for cash to meet their needs for things such as soap, oil, candles, school fees, shoes, and money for transportation to the clinic or hospital.

'M'e Masello's house exemplifies the tension between material possessions and presumed wealth while highlighting the role of memory in the material. When I met her in 2007, this 77-year-old grandmother lived with six maternal grandchildren and one paternal grandchild, ranging in age from two to 16, all orphaned by AIDS. 'M'e Masello was ill herself with chronic asthma and arthri-tis, for which she had been hospitalized several times and from which she died in 2010. She had had two houses, but one had collapsed a year before I met her, and it had yet to be rebuilt. The rocks and caved-in thatched roof lay in a heap (figure 1.7) next to the remaining rondavel, which was also in need of repair.

After the first house collapsed, 'M'e Masello moved all her possessions into the remaining home, creating extremely close quarters for the eight people liv-ing there. Inside her house, she had one metal bed frame and mattress, where she slept with the youngest child, Lebo. Next to that stood a bookshelf with an incom-plete tea set and a broken clock, an old chest, a small wooden table, blankets, mats, dishes, and containers for food and clothing. She said that her deceased husband used to give her money, but now she struggled to buy basic necessities.

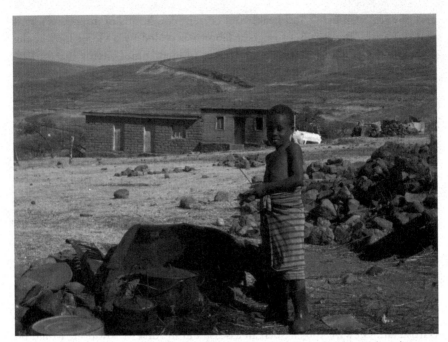

FIGURE 1.7. 'M'e Masello's grandson cooking in front of a collapsed rondavel (right), 2009

Even with the blankets folded and the sleeping mats leaning against the wall during the day, the house was cramped. The hands of the clock would never turn again, and the teacups lay in dusty chipped desuetude, yet 'M'e Masello refused to part with these items. They were a source of pride and an important connection to her late husband's memory and labor. Objects help maintain the presence of ancestral people and in many cases are sheltered in the very houses the ancestors built. During my most recent visit, I walked past 'M'e Masello's house. All its occupants had left, and it stood empty and deteriorated—a ruined monument to the social lives and objects it once contained (figure 1.8).

In the shadow of these remnants of gold-mining prosperity lie the signs of AIDS-related change on the household. Among household members' belongings are the material signs of an increasing number of interdependent children and adults. Bedrolls are tucked into corners, plastic buckets are filled with children's clothes to be washed, black school notebooks with red trim sit in neat stacks, and a pile of school uniforms await mending. These subtle signs of care are integrated with more obvious indicators of the impact of AIDS on the house. Small dirty boxes filled with pill bottles and liquids sit undisturbed until 7 a.m., when sunrise or a battery-powered clock tells the family it is time for antiretroviral medicines to be handed out. Calendars depict a red AIDS ribbon emblazoned over a picture of a mother and child or a cartoon picture of an

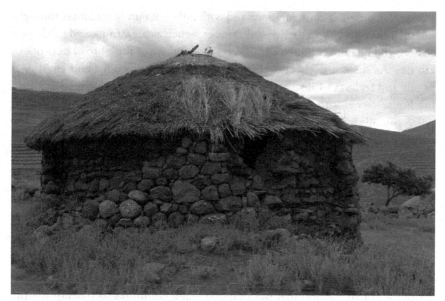

FIGURE 1.8. 'M'e Masello's unoccupied house, 2015

anthropomorphic condom. Religious items like bibles, crosses, and rosaries are tucked into corners. A near-empty sack of maize meal with the blue World Food Program symbol sits on the ground. Many of these items symbolize poverty and illness—while at the same time denoting the intensive labor of care.

AIDS has intensified the importance of the house as a space where care takes place. Routine daily care is punctuated by the complexities and challenges of caring for a child with acute HIV or associated opportunistic illnesses. AIDS has compressed the space of the house, intensifying its role in structuring care and absorbing the pressure of AIDS-related mortality and migration. The coresidential household unit is increasingly the locus of daily acts of care, which strengthen and shape relatedness. As the pressures and burdens of HIV weigh more heavily on communities and as economic opportunities—especially for migrant workers—continue to diminish, these sites of caregiving become increasingly important to the broad landscape of kinship networks in southern Africa. I explore this care in depth and detail in chapters 3 and 4.

## CONCLUSION: THE SOCIAL GEOGRAPHY OF CARE

In the midst of increasing levels of marital instability, strained relations between women and their affinal kin, the changing role of lineality, and a de-emphasis on the practice of bridewealth exchange, the house has emerged as the most stable element connecting Basotho. The house is a key crossroads where Basotho intersect in different configurations and with different family members throughout their lives. It is a space where substances—such as breastmilk and food—are shared, and it is the central locus of caregiving practices for a broad network of kin ties. As such, it is also the site where physical connections and emotional bonds and feelings of love and affection are nurtured. With this new focus on the house comes a focus on care. While investigating caregiving practices for AIDS patients in Botswana, Klaits found that activities taking place in the house "shape people's sense of the possibilities that they will receive love and care from others" (2010, 126). Care has always been an important element in Basotho relationships. The social expectation of care within the house helps maintain the house as a space where care is enacted. Likewise, a lack of care leads to the dissolution of relationships and households. Whereas the act of caring has always been emphasized as a valued characteristic of Basotho social life, as evidenced by fostering practices and respect and care for the elderly, the practical de-emphasis on markers of lineality has made care one of the primary organizing principles of the house and thus of Basotho social life. Care is no longer merely a valued social act but a primary action that has changed—and continues to transform—the social geography of rural Lesotho.

This refocus on the house, which is newly organized around caregiving, has important implications for the care of AIDS orphans. The house is a space where people can seek help and care from kin, something that is increasingly important as the number of sick and orphaned Basotho remains high. Rural communities in Lesotho are reorganizing themselves in ways that privilege care. This is possible because of the flexibility and fluidity of kinship, the disconnect that exists between idealized notions of kinship and patrilineality, and the realities of everyday practice. It is common for Basotho to live in households composed of various members from either side of the family. Likewise, children are accustomed to movement between households for both material and emotional reasons. A flexible understanding of relatedness allows Basotho to cement bonds among a range of kin in order to expand networks of care when families are in need.

The testaments of many of the caregivers I got to know well indicate that some of the things that are threatening the unity of the family are also helping ensure that children are not left without care. First, there is the strong—almost self-evident—belief that orphaned children should remain within the extended family. The rural and close-knit nature of the villages surrounding the camptown of Mokhotlong, as well as the virtual absence of institutional facilities, means that families rarely consider options for care outside of the family unit. Unifying practices such as bridewealth payments are occurring with much less frequency and consistency. This appears to be weakening the connections between affinal kin, reducing the incentive for parents of a married couple to intervene and prevent a separation or divorce so as to maintain ties between clans. However, while bridewealth has declined in practice, it remains an important cultural ideal and marker of lineality in Lesotho. This gap between ideal and practice creates a space where the rules of Sesotho kinship can be negotiated to provide the best possible situation for children (see chapter 4). And while children born to HIV-positive mothers face insecurity, due to the mother's compromised health and their own potentially compromised health, the support network has not collapsed. The affection for children and their general cultural significance have helped maintain a strong commitment to caring for them within the extended family network, ensuring their protection even after their parents have died. The resulting negotiations for the care of AIDS orphans are then centered on the house as the central space where Basotho kinship is enacted. The house provides a stable measure of kinship practices and relatedness even as other aspects of Basotho kinship ebb and flow.

# 2 · MEDICAL PLURALISM IN A LOW-RESOURCE SETTING

## The Sesotho Doctors

*It is late Friday afternoon, knock-off time, and the main road is lined with pedestrians three abreast. Men and women saunter toward the weekend, yelling at neighbors across the road, laughing, aiming for warm meals and soft chairs. Beside us, taxis glide in slo-mo. Mokhotlong's fleet of battered four-plus-ones are on the prowl this afternoon, drivers honking as they pass potential fares, arms out the windows—"Uena, u ea kae, where you going?" Then the wind picks up, and everyone on the road turns in unison—we shield ourselves from the rolling wall of dust—and all around us tarps strung over shanties snap and pop in the wind.*

*A man crosses the street, heading for me.*

*"My brother, can we just talk?"*

*He's dressed in all white: white hat, white jacket, white slacks, white beaded necklace, black turtleneck—no one really dresses in all white after all—the man's no fool. He's sporting leather boots that come to wicked metal tips, and he's got a scar running from his right temple, by the hairline, to the peak of his cheekbone: a serious scar, businesslike and efficient, no jagged detours or Baroque curvature—just a straight angry slice.*

*"I'm a Sesotho doctor, ngaka ea Sesotho, professionally trained. My brother, I'm selling medicine."*

*He holds up a red plastic pail that once contained individually wrapped pieces of bubble gum. Dark liquid sloshes inside.*

*"My medicine cures many ailments," the man tells me, slipping into a well-worn salesman's cadence.*

*He holds up his pinkie finger: "High blood."*

*Up goes the ring finger: "Frustration."*

*Now the middle finger: "Even these STDs."*

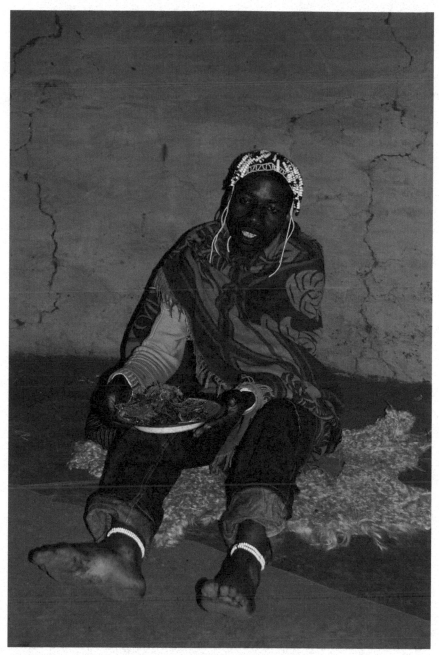

FIGURE 2.1. Sesotho doctor from Mokhotlong with medicinal plants, 2018 (Photo by Nastassia Donoho, reprinted with permission.)

He holds up a forth finger, then changes course. "The body is full of cells—that's what this medicine is for. It cleans the blood, cleans the cells."

I ask him what it's made from—is it natural?

"Yes, it's natural medicine. It's English medicine and Sesotho medicine together. Powerful medicine but more powerful for Basotho people."

I want to ask him more about this—Can medicine really work differently for people of different cultures?—but I'm in a hurry right now, with no time to buy medicine and no time for philosophical inquiry. I'm rushing toward Nurse Seeng's office. Ellen and I are heading to Namibia soon, and I need to pick up malaria medicine for our kids before the nurse closes up for the weekend.

The Sesotho doctor doesn't seem overly concerned that I'm not buying. "Come see me again," he says. "We can talk more on Monday."

This Sesotho doctor is from Quthing—on the opposite side of the country—and he is new to the area. Perhaps this is why he is out in the street hustling for customers. Most practitioners of Sesotho medicine set up shop in the metal shanties along the main road, where they can build a client base.

Down the road a bit, for instance, is the shop of Ntate Leseko, who has been practicing Sesotho medicine for more than 30 years. I went to visit him one afternoon, an older man with a long and neatly trimmed beard, always dressed in church clothes: a collared shirt under a sweater, fancy slacks, and dark polished shoes. You might mistake him for an accountant if not for the fox pelts hanging outside his shop, a cramped shanty, warmly redolent of incense oil. Inside, he keeps his Sesotho medicines arranged fastidiously in shoeboxes, each ingredient filed away on a shelf. Thirty boxes maybe, each with a handwritten label: tlapi, tsitabaloi, hloenya, sefaha, phela, double cheek. The ingredients poke over the tops of the containers—I can see tangles of twigs, roots and bark, and dried leaves. Ntate Leseko says he learned his trade from a Malawian man who showed him where to dig for these items, then picked up more natural medicine from some Zulu men he visits on business trips. Sometimes he'll close up shop for a week or more to forage for plants and supplies, traveling as far as the South African provinces of KwaZulu-Natal or Gauteng.

Ntate Leseko says he can cure many ailments: "If they have sores on their private parts or spinal cord pain, things like headache and stomachache and all the illnesses of the body. If someone wants me to phatsa, to use the razor to cut them and apply medicine, I can do it." He stops for a moment. "Sometimes they have a mental problem and need me to phatsa so the medicine can enter their blood."

Even HIV falls within the purview of Ntate Leseko's medical treatment. "There is a Sesotho medicine to help it," he says, "but now it is gone. I found it only in Natal—green in color and when you taste it, it tastes like chili." But while he is sure of his craft, the doctor admits that sometimes Sesotho medicine can work even better in concert with Western treatments. For HIV, he gives patients this plant from KwaZulu-Natal and then instructs them to take "the English pills" too.

He tells a story about an HIV-positive man he was treating with Sesotho medicine. Everything was going well, he says, but the man's son told his father to stop using Sesotho medicine and go instead to the hospital. Here Ntate Leseko grows frustrated: "When I was working with him, the man was not becoming more sick—but he went to the hospital and got the pills, and then he became more sick! He was very sick, and he was very angry with his child."

The doctor sighs and watches the pedestrian traffic outside his shop: "But I have seen people being better when they start with my Sesotho medicine and then go to the hospital. Sometimes they can be good together—the Sesotho medicine and the English medicine."

'M'e Malelang disagrees; she doesn't trust English medicine. She is another ngaka ea Sesotho, a competitor to Ntate Leseko, with a stand across the street. Her wares are laid out on a table, less ordered and meticulous than her rival but perhaps more likely to entice window shoppers. In her braids she wears the traditional beads that Sesotho doctors sometimes favor, and a small goat horn hangs from a band around her neck. 'M'e Malelang told Ellen that she became a Sesotho doctor because of a dream. "I was having moea," 'M'e Malelang says, using a Sesotho word that means wind or spirit, a word that refers to the visions that Sesotho doctors sometimes experience. "I saw these in my dream"—she is touching the beads in her hair—"I saw the ngaka ea Sesotho, so I went to him, and he trained me for a week. Later, other things were shown to me by the ancestors."

Mostly she treats children—even Sesotho doctors must have their specialties—but 'M'e Malelang says she can cure HIV as well. Then she backtracks: "Actually, I don't believe that infection is even there."

Ellen pauses, then asks what is responsible for the deaths that have been ravaging the country for years now.

"Kannete, I don't know," she says, "but I don't believe that infection exists—it is other illnesses."

'M'e Malelang stops for a moment, grows quiet.

"Once, even I went to those English doctors. Do you know what they told me? They tested me and said I had AIDS."

'M'e Malelang's voice is measured as she continues.

"But I didn't use their pills. And now I have cured myself with Sesotho medicine."

* * *

I've reached Nurse Seeng's office just in time, and she laughs as I hustle through the door, telling me to rest easy. Some months back, our kids treated her to an impromptu dance performance—tumbling and stunting in her office, jitterbugging through the room—and she asks after them now: Where are my angels? Where are my darlings?

Nurse Seeng brings out the malaria meds, and we chat for a moment about the upcoming trip. Then I tell her about the Sesotho doctor I met earlier along the road.

She is a Mosotho woman—and someone whose grandfather was a Sesotho doctor himself—but she is trained in Western medicine. She has built and funded this clinic by herself and has earned herself a thriving business. She has more work than she can handle—the town hungry for someone of her skills, her demeanor, and her patience and compassion—and shorter wait times than the district hospital. So I am curious what she, from her cultural vantage, has to say about Sesotho medicine.

"Hmm," she says, still smiling. "I suppose those herbs do have some efficacy."

Nurse Seeng is slow to speak ill of anyone, but a note of skepticism begins to slip into her voice.

"And while those herbs can provide relief, I do have some questions. How do those Sesotho doctors know the right dosages? Are those plants tested and measured? Do they have contaminants, micro-organisms—are they safely prepared?"

Nurse Seeng smiles again and places her hands on her desk. "As for the people who are treated—I think we can say that people are healed by what they believe. If someone believes in the power of these herbs, then they will believe the herbs have cured them—they will truly believe they feel better."

Then her voice cools.

"But where is the proof? Can it be proved beyond just words?"

She stops again, and her eyes narrow.

"And you know that some of these Sesotho 'doctors' are doing this work only for money. They can give people any kind of plant and claim it is medicine. They don't care if it works."

Now Nurse Seeng's voice takes on an edge that I've never heard from her before.

"Do you want to know the worst thing? Some people believe they have been bewitched. When they have HIV, they say they have been bewitched, and they will never go to a doctor who knows English medicine. They will never. And then people die who could have been helped."

She sits back in her seat.

"Really—it is pathetic."

\* \* \*

Back on the main road and heading home.

As I walk, I pass tables and stands spread with Sesotho medicine. It has been a few years now since Ellen and I spoke with Ntate Leseko and 'M'e Malelang. A friend recently told me that Ntate Leseko's son has gone into pharmacy school at the university in Roma. What must the boy's father think of this? Is he proud that his son is carrying on the family trade? Disappointed that his boy has rejected the old ways? Or perhaps Ntate Leseko sees it as some complicated navigation of traditions?

Further along the road, I pass another Sesotho doctor. I stop to talk for a moment, but we are having difficulty communicating—neither his English nor my Sesotho are *strong enough to bridge the gap. But before I leave, I ask if he knows 'M'e Malelang. Does he know if she is still in town? It's been a while since I've seen her.*

*He rolls the name around in his mouth, trying to untangle meaning from my accent. Then comprehension dawns. He says her name again—slowly, clearly—wants to make sure he's got it right. I nod.*

*He says something quickly in Sesotho. I can't catch his meaning, so I ask again—Is she still here?*

*The man shakes his head—Ah ah—points a finger toward the sky.*

-WM-

\* \* \*

## SEEKING TREATMENT, SEEKING CARE

The subject of this book is kinship and the ways that families and communities have responded to the AIDS crisis. But it is set in one of the poorest regions in southern Africa, and so it is also fundamentally about how poverty, inequality, and disease are entangled with kinship. In this chapter, I consider how Basotho make choices about their health—navigating a world of biomedical doctors and indigenous healers—and demonstrate how treatment-seeking decisions are localized, culturally produced responses to poverty and structural inequality. I also show how even in (or perhaps, especially in) resource-poor contexts, people make medical decisions that protect their social relations, even at the cost of their own health.

Culture is a complex web of beliefs, norms, and practices, not merely a byproduct of social structures. Most attempts to define culture are so vast that they almost cease to be meaningful. Yet culture, while powerful, is constrained by structures that make certain options feasible, rational, or inevitable. The anthropological affinity for culture and for emphasizing the importance of cultural relativism can get in the way of recognizing that beliefs and practices often emerge in response to poverty and inequality. As Paul Farmer bluntly puts it, anthropologists have had the tendency "to confuse structural violence with cultural difference" (2009, 23). Furthermore, he argues, "Awareness of cultural differences has long complicated discussion of human suffering" (2009, 23). Likewise, Julie Taylor warns that although culture can be a useful concept to employ, we need to be "aware of its subordinating potential" (2007, 974). With our particular attention to culture in addressing HIV/AIDS, Taylor argues, "anthropologists, often unawares, collude with and facilitate the creation of difference, and thus the hegemonic exercise of power" (2007, 974). In other words, an overemphasis on cultural difference can act like a smoke screen, drawing attention away from the unequal structures and power differences that produce suffering, absolving distant observers from any complicity in it. This strategy is evident in the emphasis in HIV research on culturally specific sexual and health behaviors—such as multiple concurrent partnerships and poor adherence to medication—which present the spread of HIV as inevitable due to deeply rooted (and deviant) cultural practices. I argue that health care structures both limit and shape therapeutic possibilities but also that culture works within those powerful structures. Medical pluralism in Mokhotlong, I suggest, is a cultural response to structural conditions. Rural Basotho's ideas about biomedicine and indigenous healing are a response to history, disease trajectories, and a chronic lack of resources. And while therapies, policies, and resources shift, families remain ever present even as they change and adapt to structural conditions.

Most people in Mokhotlong view illness and select treatment approaches based on culturally mediated understandings of several seemingly rigid binaries: biomedical causality versus nonbiomedical causality, symptom management versus disease management, and "English" medicine versus Sesotho medicine. However, Basotho negotiate these binaries by employing culturally salient strategies to address health problems that are often produced and constrained by poverty. Patients and caregivers draw on these malleable resources in order to make choices that consider both the physical and social implications of their actions. This flexibility allows them to navigate complex situations with few resources while simultaneously protecting networks of kinship and care.

Basotho's choices about treatments—and the underlying explanatory models of health and illness that stem from them—implicate the realm of kin and care. Here, as elsewhere, social relationships are enmeshed with biomedical knowledge about disease transmission and etiology. As biomedical treatments become increasingly available, they are favored by a growing number of Basotho precisely because they help protect the health of loved ones. Ultimately, the ethnographic data regarding pluralistic treatment seeking and the conceptions of illness, as I present them here, serve to elucidate Basotho responses to HIV and reinforce the notion that AIDS is a kinship disease. Yet these same data also highlight how kinship ideals and practices are fundamentally limited and shaped by poverty and inequality.

## LESOTHO'S HEALTH CARE SYSTEM: STRUCTURE AND FUNDING

Before presenting an in-depth exploration of the ways in which people negotiate the medical landscape in Lesotho, it is important to establish the choices that are available. Basotho's navigation of the seemingly rigid binaries concerning medical treatment and disease etiologies does not exist in a vacuum. Rather, structural and social inequalities constrain treatment choices, and Basotho's decisions and their understandings of illness and treatment must be viewed within this context. Rural Basotho have limited access to health care facilities. Debilitating poverty, a lack of transport, and weather conditions that frequently constrain travel to and from the clinic all inhibit patients' ability to show up at a medical facility. Once there, overworked and undertrained medical personnel are often unable to provide high-quality care. In this section, I examine the broad structure of Lesotho's health and social welfare system, describe biomedical health care options available for Basotho living in the Mokhotlong district, and briefly examine how other social services and NGOs support their health and welfare.

The ministry of health and social welfare coordinates government medical services in all 10 districts of Lesotho. These are supplemented by numerous private organizations, most notably the Christian Health Association of Lesotho (CHAL),[1] Baylor International Pediatric AIDS Initiative (BIPAI), Médecins Sans Frontières (MSF), and Partners in Health (PIH), which, at times, have funded and run hospitals and clinics throughout the country. According to the ministry website, there are 22 public and private hospitals in Lesotho (Lesotho Ministry of Health 2011). The district of Maseru, with the country's highest population concentration and where the capital city is located, has seven hospitals and the highest number of public and private clinics and receives patients from throughout the country who need specialized care or complex surgery. All other districts have either one or two hospitals and an average of 15 public clinics and a few private clinics (see table 2.1).

Despite a seemingly large number of health facilities, there is an acute human-resource shortage in the health care sector. According to the WHO (World Health Organization; 2006), Lesotho had a density of health care providers

TABLE 2.1. Distribution of hospitals and clinics in Lesotho

| District | Population | Hospitals | Clinics (public) | Clinics (private) |
|---|---|---|---|---|
| Maseru | 477,599 | 7 (incl. 2 specialty) | 49 | 70 percent of country's private practitioners |
| Berea | 300,557 | 2 | 12 | 4 |
| Leribe | 362,339 | 2 | 31 | 5 |
| Buthe-Buthe | 126,948 | 2 | 10 | 3 |
| Mokhotlong | 89,705 | 1 | 10 | 1 |
| Qacha's Nek | 80,323 | 2 | 12 | 1 |
| Thaba-Tseka | 133,680 | 2 | 20 | 3 |
| Quthing | 140,641 | 2 | 9 | 1 |
| Mohale's Hoek | 206,842 | 1 | 12 | 3 |
| Mafeteng | 238,946 | 1 | 19 | 3 |

SOURCE: Lesotho Ministry of Health (2011).

(including doctors, nurses, and midwives) of only 1.15 per 1,000 patients. The WHO-recommended threshold for the density of health care providers is 2.3 per 1,000. At the time of this report—2006—only 89 doctors and 1,123 nurses and midwives were working in Lesotho, and the workforce was young, which is problematic for training and mentorship (WHO 2006). A decade later, little had changed. Many of the doctors I knew in Mokhotlong were from places like Sierra Leone and Zimbabwe, countries with good universities but a history of conflict that drove out educated elites.[2] Most saw their posts in Lesotho as temporary until they could find higher-paying jobs in other parts of southern Africa or as an immigration strategy to get them to their final destinations: South Africa, the United Kingdom, or sometimes Canada. MSF supported 14 clinics, and in 2007, half of the nurse posts at these clinics were vacant, as were more than 30 percent of nursing posts at the district hospital in the region in which they were working (Médecins Sans Frontières 2007). The ethnography in this chapter frequently presents an overworked and at times seemingly uncaring medical staff. These encounters must be read in a context where the rewards, upward mobility, and compensation for work do not match the physically and emotionally exhausting workload and where the lack of resources lead to dishearteningly poor patient outcomes.

When seeking medical care in Lesotho, the courses of action a patient can take are influenced by a complex combination of factors, including cost, proximity, and available treatment. At the hospital, patients pay a nominal fee for an outpatient visit: only 15 Maloti (approximately $1.20), including treatment and medication. Treatment at government and CHAL clinics is free, but some medications are not. Private clinics are the most expensive—the base price of a visit is 150 Maloti ($12)—and are typically used by wealthier Basotho, but in Mokhotlong, the diagnostic tests and treatments available in these clinics cost extra and are often only marginally better than those available at public facilities. In a private clinic, however, a patient can expect to spend more time with the provider, lines are shorter, and supplies are more consistently available. For specialized care or the most up-to-date medical technologies (including any kind of oncology), those who can afford to do so travel to South Africa.

Clinics can provide basic outpatient services and medications, subject to availability, including antibiotics, immunizations, HIV testing, ART (antiretroviral therapy), antenatal care, and well-baby care. However, patients need to go to a hospital for inpatient care, IV fluids, minor surgeries, and certain tests that require lab work or specialized machinery, such as X-rays and liver-function tests. A motorcycle courier service collects blood samples for TB (tuberculosis) and CD4 (cluster of differentiation 4) counts from the clinics and brings them to the district hospitals within a few hours of being drawn. However, rural TB patients in need of chest X-rays must make the trip to the hospital located in each district's central town (or camptown), which can be expensive and time consuming, often involving a day of travel, a day in line at the hospital, and a day's return travel.

The majority of people in the Mokhotlong district use the government-run hospitals and clinics or CHAL clinics, although they occasionally pay to go to the private clinic for anonymity, speed, and quality of service—or a second opinion. At the district hospital, one is likely to wait a half-day to see the doctor plus another half-day to collect medications from the pharmacy. A visit to a private clinic takes an hour. Since 2004, ARVs (antiretroviral drugs) have been free in Lesotho, supported largely by the U.S.-government-funded program PEPFAR (President's Emergency Plan for AIDS Relief) and by the Global Fund (funded by the Gates Foundation). The government has been expanding access to treatment, clinic by clinic, across the country. ARVs were first available at select clinics and hospitals, then at government clinics located closest to the camptowns, and finally at clinics farther from population centers. This was a slow but essential development in improving access to treatment for those living in the most remote villages. At the Mokhotlong Hospital, ART patients skip the main outpatient building and walk up the hill to the very back of the hospital property, where the Lerato Center is discreetly located (*lerato* is Sesotho for "love"). There they have their monthly ART appointment, where their adherence is monitored by counting leftover pills, medications are refilled, and any other problems are addressed. In the rural clinics, one day per week is dedicated to treating ART patients only. On this day, patients receive all necessary medications, but still, certain diagnostic tests require them to travel to the hospital for care.

In addition to these public and private health services, numerous local and international NGOs work throughout Lesotho in an attempt to address the peripheral impacts of HIV. It is impossible to generalize about the function and efficacy of these organizations. The term *NGO* has come to signify a panoply of groups: religious organizations, those working in capacities that otherwise would have been filled by civil society, and those working against local elite institutions and practices (Fisher 1997). NGOs often pick up the slack in the absence of effective state resources but at a social and political cost. As Kenworthy (2017) explains in her ethnography of the scale up of programs and organizations that attempt to address the ravages of AIDS in Lesotho, these services are wildly uneven, notoriously difficult to navigate, and have contributed to depoliticization and social unrest.

In addition to the variety of social services provided by NGOs working in Lesotho, the department of social welfare, a subsidiary of the ministry of health and social welfare, has some resources to provide social supports to orphans and vulnerable children. However, social work has historically been an undervalued and underfunded profession in Lesotho, with the first cohort of locally trained social workers graduating from the National University of Lesotho in 2005 (Chitereka 2009). As of 2013, only 200 social workers were employed in the country, and they were not managed or trained by any one regulatory body (Tanga 2013). In the Mokhotlong district, there was one social worker at the local hospital: 'M'e Linda. I tried on numerous occasions to meet with her, but she was never available by phone. I stopped by her office several times, and although she was often sitting at her desk, she always told me to come back another time. I later learned that she and some of the MCS (Mokhotlong Children's Services) staff were not on good terms, which is perhaps why she refused to speak with me. Many caregivers I spoke with said that they had heard that they could receive services from social workers through the social welfare office by registering the orphans in their care, but none succeeded in doing so. Most caregivers simply said that there were no social workers to help them, likely a reflection of the complete lack of funding and training for social workers. Instead, they cobbled together services and support from a variety of sources, including a few locally based NGOs like MCS. Many received food from the World Food Program, and some were savvy (or lucky) in gaining the support of the other international NGOs that came and went from Mokhotlong. In addition to these biomedical treatment options, many Mokhotlong residents continued to seek care from indigenous healers or Sesotho doctors. I will present these treatment-seeking strategies in the following section.

## BIOMEDICAL AND NONBIOMEDICAL DISEASE ETIOLOGIES

In 2017, Tumo, 'M'e Nthabiseng's 22-year-old son, spent a few months living with us in Minnesota while on a break from university in South Africa. Tumo was prone to sleeping in, and we were surprised to find him up early one morning, standing in his pajamas at the kettle, waiting for water to boil. Will overheard him talking to our five-year-old daughter, Eve, who was interrogating him about why he was up so early. He told her, "I think I'm starting to feel the beginning of a cold." "Yeah, I had a cold too," Eve replied. "I got it from Mara," she continued, pinning the cold's provenance on her perpetually stuffed-up nine-month-old sister, who at that moment had a steady stream of snot running from her nose. Tumo jumped to the baby's defense: "I think it might just be the weather. We don't have to put it on Mara." In many conversations I had, Basotho were hesitant to acknowledge the ways in which infections spread between people, due to the threat this could pose to tight-knit social relationships. Instead, Tumo offered a generalized and impersonal explanation for his cold. While this conversation between Tumo and Eve was innocuous given the illness involved, the acknowledgment of person-to-person transmission of HIV between sexual partners and from mother to child presents real threats to social networks of kinship and care.

After many fieldwork conversations and a few ethnographic gaffes—where I asked potentially painful finger-pointing questions about disease transmission—I realized that Basotho caregivers usually discussed the causality of disease in a way that best protected their networks of kin and care. Disease etiologies lie at the confluence of limited, cost-prohibitive treatment options and cultural ideas about disease that are in line with Basotho's relational orientation to the world. Conceptions about the origins of illness were at once scientific and speculative; they derived from an understanding that illness could have both natural and supernatural causes. A single person might provide a range of explanations for an illness—simultaneously including God, witches, and airborne transmission. Kwansa (2014) found this to be true in Ghana as well, where people looked for spiritual causes and sought spiritual healing for HIV while still also taking their ARVs. Although Basotho sometimes mentioned an illness spreading from person to person in an abstract way, they rarely expounded on the details. Yet as the examples that follow demonstrate, patients are comfortable with the contradictions that arise between these beliefs and their treatment-seeking behaviors. Most patients I encountered did not see multiple etiological explanations as being mutually exclusive, and many were comfortable with a lack of clarity about cause. As with Tumo's refusal to blame his cold on baby Mara, this flexibility was not born out of ignorance but rather used as a resource to protect both health and social networks, particularly when effective treatments were unavailable, unaffordable, or otherwise structurally constrained. One of the primary ways that Basotho avoided placing blame on loved ones was to focus on divine causes of illness, even as the biological ones were well known.

Christian churches in southern Africa are appealing to local populations due to their healing powers (Klaits 2010; Comaroff 1985; Janzen 1992),[3] and religious institutions have been heavily involved in both the spiritual and the biomedical aspects of HIV treatment and healing (Dilger, Burchardt, and van Dijk 2014). Dilger and his colleagues argue that it is impossible to look at HIV treatment outside of the "social and moral" priorities of religious organizations (2014, 14). The need for both physical and spiritual healing has reopened a new space for churches in this regard, particularly for people living with HIV. These healing-focused "churches of the spirit" have an appeal "based on bringing participants' sentiments to bear on one another's bodies in ways that enhance well-being" (Klaits 2010, 8). The majority of Basotho are affiliated with some branch of Christianity; in 2014, only 2 percent of women and 8 percent of men did not so associate (Lesotho Ministry of Health 2016). Though a relatively small community, Mokhotlong has dozens of Christian churches of all denominations and sizes, some of which are focused on faith healing. While some congregations gather in large permanent stone structures, others meet weekly in tents out by the airstrip or in tin shacks nestled anonymously into neighborhoods, recognizable on Sundays by the chorus of voices and the strains of synthesizer gospel hymns floating out into the day.

Despite discouragement from their Christian religious leaders, many Basotho also maintain beliefs in non-Christian spiritual forces, such as witchcraft. For the most part, the churches ignore these kinds of heterodox beliefs, though in some cases, certain behaviors are reprimanded. For example, if a young person chooses to participate in the three-month-long initiation school that is a traditional rite of passage into adulthood, they may have to do community-service hours for their church as punishment. However, these mild repercussions do not dissuade people from following certain aspects of what many refer to simply as "Sesotho culture" while also allowing churches to maintain at least the semblance of authority over spiritual affairs. Even the Sesotho doctor Ntate Leseko told me that he believed in God and thought God was instrumental in helping him with his work. However, his work as a Sesotho doctor did limit his ability to practice his Christian faith. When I asked him if he attended church, he replied, "No, now I don't. The problem is the church that I was attending doesn't go with the medicines. And I am meant to use the medicines. And I'm not able to go to church because of that. My children are attending that church. And their mother has passed away, and she was still attending that church." Despite the resulting alienation from his chosen place of worship, Ntate Leseko viewed his profession as a calling, one that even faith in God could not alter.

Basotho believers often draw on their Christian faith to explain the origins of their illnesses or to come to terms with their suffering. 'M'e Maliehi, an observant Catholic (*Roma*), wondered about the possible connections between illness and God: "*Ntate-Molimo* [God the Father]? [*laughs*] *Ache*, I don't know. Maybe he is the one because everything is provided by him." When asked about the cause of her granddaughter's albinism, one woman claimed there was no explanation: "No one knows how one becomes albino . . . I don't know, it is God who makes that." However, natural causality does not preclude divine causality, and vice versa. Basotho understand and explain illness by invoking God even while acknowledging that the immediate cause might be something more mundane.

In the following conversation, 'M'e Masello insisted that God was the only cause of HIV and therefore the only cure, but at the end of the conversation, she admitted to the importance of taking ARVs. When I asked her where sickness came from, she said, "It's how God has provided it" and then went on to explain original sin by summarizing the story of Adam and Eve. Ausi Ntsoaki, my research assistant, tried to get to a more proximal cause by asking, "Are we infected by other people, or do we take it from the air, or we eat from food or witches or spirits?" 'M'e Masello refused to answer. Instead, she offered the following insight: "Ha ha, God has provided illness. We will not find only the good things from him. We can run to the doctors, but if God doesn't want us to be cured, we won't be cured. But if God raises up his hand, we will be cured." I wanted to know how this worked in a practical sense, so I asked her if God could cure HIV or provide ARVs. She told me, "They are still doing them [ARVs], those who are doing them. And they are cured, and they become fat. AIDS patients, they go there when they are not able to walk, being taken by wheelchairs. And they are given only those pills and a lot of food." In 'M'e Masello's mind, I was imposing a false dichotomy on the scenario: she believed fully in God's omnipotence yet was also aware of the transformative powers of ARVs, which she witnessed working on her own grandson, Lebo. For 'M'e Masello, dwelling on the spiritual origins of illness was socially powerful, something that did not negatively impact her grandson's health or treatment in any way. This strategy also worked as a bridge for 'M'e Masello, addressing the gaps left by poverty and by the unequal global distribution of disease, which makes the best treatments unavailable to the world's poor.

Basotho are much better informed about HIV/AIDS than they were in the early 2000s. Yet in the context of the high AIDS death rate in Lesotho and with limited treatment options, an acceptance of the unknowable and a lack of attention to actual modes of transmission allow family members to circumvent the implications of sexual and mother-to-child transmission. I am embarrassed to recall how—when I was just beginning my fieldwork—I asked the caregivers of HIV-positive children if they knew how the children had become infected. My goal at the time was to assess levels of HIV knowledge, and I was dismayed by what seemed like a lack of information in this area. I later realized that giving voice to this answer would mean acknowledging that one family member had infected another with HIV. When I asked 'M'e Mamorena if she knew how Hopolang was infected, she quickly answered no. I asked if she had any guesses, and again she replied no. However, when I asked if she thought the girl got it from her mother, she said, "Yes, I think so, because I said the child was very young, and she was in the stomach [of her mother]. How has she gotten this? I was asking [myself], 'Has she gotten this from her mother?' And other people who were coming to see her said she has gotten it from her mother. Ache, Hopolang . . . she was so sick." When pressed, people could talk in more detail about biomedical disease etiologies—but they often preferred not to do so. I abandoned this line of questioning as soon as I realized that I was forcing caregivers to voice knowledge that compromised both the memory of their deceased loved ones and their caregiving relationships.

Dwelling on the modes of transmission would place the blame on mothers for infecting children and spouses for infecting their partners. These husbands, wives, and mothers will likely be called on to care for—or be cared for by—these same family members. Although it might help prevent the future transmission of disease, a focus on transmission creates tension between family members, adding to the caregiver's burden. With a high AIDS mortality rate and during a time when infants regularly become sick and die, faith in God reinforces an essential access point of understanding and solace for many Basotho. A spiritual etiology of HIV can also explain why ARVs help some people on the brink of death while others perish or why some mothers infect their children during labor or breast-feeding while others do not. Biomedical explanations frequently do not have the capacity to elucidate differential patient outcomes and resiliencies, leaving the painful ways that AIDS alters the family unaddressed and unresolved.

In some ways, Basotho's syncretic understanding of disease etiology is the binary least impacted by structural inequalities, at least in terms of treatment-seeking behaviors. However, if all the resources that are available to AIDS patients in the Global North were also available in Lesotho, the epidemiological landscape would be vastly different, obviating the need to protect loved ones by obfuscating biomedical realities.

## MANAGING SYMPTOMS, MANAGING DISEASE

Like the seeming contrast between biomedical and nonbiomedical conceptions of disease, Basotho in rural Mokhotlong also navigate another "binary": symptom management versus disease management. Just as the emphasis on spiritual causes of disease draws attention away from modes of contraction and blame and protects the relationship between the caregiver and care receiver, the emphasis on outward symptoms of disease in Mokhotlong also has a strategic element. In Lesotho, HIV treatment is fundamentally shaped and limited by structural inequalities. Basotho responses to HIV/AIDS must then focus on mediating the social and relational consequences of the illness in creative ways while address-ing the physical illness. When I first began my fieldwork, it seemed as though Basotho only acknowledged the outward manifestations of illness, and this could create significant challenges for treating HIV, which requires that a patient take ARVs for life, regardless of symptoms. Basotho patients and caregivers tended to focus on locally salient symptoms of AIDS, as elsewhere in Africa (Chimwaza and Watkins 2004; Liddell, Barrett, and Bydawell 2005). However, if the focus on symptoms were to play out to its logical conclusion, one might expect to find poor rates of adherence to ARVs once a patient's viral load had recovered and an outward appearance of "health" returned. However, studies have demonstrated high levels of adherence to ART in African settings (Mills et al. 2006; Nachega et al. 2004), and the focus on symptom management has not been a significant factor in influencing adherence to treatment (Bhengu et al. 2011).

Many caregivers emphasized symptoms, such as rashes and diarrhea, rather than the underlying indicators of HIV, such as CD4 counts, yet they success-fully adhered to treatment regimens well after they experienced drastic health improvements. The focus on symptom management was not at the expense of managing the underlying disease but was a contextually selective strategy used by Basotho caregivers to balance both physical and social needs. On the one hand, a symptom-centered approach is often the only feasible approach in Mokhotlong. The observable and lived reality of illness—when multiple diagnostic tests and careful explanations of the inner workings of illness are neither possible nor expected—necessitates a reliance on the physical experiences of illness. On the other hand, a symptom-centered approach also has the benefit of drawing attention away from the underlying illness, its intimate modes of transmission, and its potential long-term outcomes so that people can continue to live future-oriented and meaningful lives. This helps remove blame and places focus on the caregiving relationship (Chimwaza and Watkins 2004), reinforcing the centrality of the caregiver's role. In a context where kin-based care is the norm and institutional care is all but nonexistent, preserving these caregiving relationships is a matter of life and death, especially for dependent children.

Health care providers in Lesotho reinforce this focus on symptom reduction. Doctors and nurses are accustomed to testing for and diagnosing a number of high-profile illnesses such as TB and HIV[4]—yet if the health care provider does not suspect one of these illnesses is present, the symptoms may be treated without further exploring the cause. In many cases, health care professionals are overworked and do not have time to make a proper diagnosis. In addition, diagnostic tests are expensive and difficult to attain due to resource and personnel shortages. One day, 'M'e Mathabelang, an outreach worker, and I took six-month-old Reitumetse to the private clinic because he had been vomiting for several days. When we told the doctor about Reitumetse's symptoms, he prescribed antibiotics, an antidiarrheal drug, an oral rehydration solution, antinausea medication, and multivitamins—an array of medications all intended to address various symptoms. He did not ask us any questions about the child's medical history or make any attempt to diagnose the underlying medical condition. Given Reitumetse's symptoms, it is likely that his vomiting was caused by a viral infection and therefore did not need antibiotic treatment. Some of the other medications prescribed also seemed unnecessary, with possible side effects that might increase the boy's nausea, particularly given how little food he was able to keep down. I expressed my concern about giving so many drugs to such a small person, but 'M'e Mathabelang was confident and undeterred. This interaction, which was viewed as a normal and effective response to Reitumetse's symptoms by both the doctor and 'M'e Mathabelang, reflects a systemic emphasis on symptom management. It also reflects the suboptimal care that often takes place in medical settings in Lesotho (see chapter 3).

Yet the focus on symptom management in Mokhotlong is rarely straightforward. 'M'e Malefu, a village health worker who had some health training, told me she often took medications only until she was able to get her symptoms under control, regardless of how long the doctor had prescribed them. She did, however, see the importance in distinguishing between different illnesses, later telling me that a patient could not stop taking their HIV or TB medications, even if the symptoms had disappeared: "If they stop them, I have seen them getting sicker. Especially TB patients. . . . No, they cannot stop them." Although some HIV and TB patients default on their medications, often due to unpleasant side effects, most Basotho understand the importance of continued biomedical treatments for certain illnesses even after symptoms have ceased. The adherence sessions that all HIV patients and caregivers are required to attend emphasize that ART is "for life." Yet structural barriers such as poverty, poor infrastructure, and distance create obstacles for adherence to ART (Hardon et al. 2007; Ncama et al. 2008; Crane et al. 2006).

People living with HIV who are not experiencing any symptoms—either because their viral load is low or because they are managing their disease effectively with ART—often avoid thinking and talking about the underlying implications and the long-term ramifications of their illness. I saw this when talking one time with 'M'e Nthabiseng, who has several HIV-infected members in her immediate family, including Lerato, a child she fostered for many years. 'M'e Nthabiseng's knowledge of HIV transmission, treatment, and prevention is extensive. She makes decisions for the health and care of hundreds of children served by MCS each year, is kept up-to-date on current research and care standards by visiting doctors, and is a certified HIV counselor and tester. She is also well aware that Lesotho has limited treatments available and that the eventual need for second-line ARVs is inevitable, even for those—like Lerato—who have near-perfect adherence. Whenever I asked her how Lerato was doing, she always assured me that she was doing well. One evening, we were at her house preparing dinner. Lerato ran into the kitchen and said, "'M'e, it's time for me to take my medicine," and proceeded to take the appropriate pills out of their little white plastic bottles and swallow them with a swig of water. As Lerato went back into the living room to join the others watching South African soap operas, I asked 'M'e Nthabiseng if she had any fears for Lerato's future. She continued to stir the *papa* with a wooden stick and said, "No, I don't have fears about her future as long as by the time she decides to leave, she's old enough to take care of herself." I then asked her if Lerato's HIV status was a cause of concern. She replied, "I don't even think about it. It's normal. I see it as normal life. It's not anything to worry about, because I could die before Lerato does, so for her to have HIV—it's not changing anything. It's a normal life. What happens happens." This minimization of the underlying disease—both for 'M'e Nthabiseng and for other caregivers—is a strategy that, while not at the expense of children's health, holds in abatement AIDS's power to destroy families. One of the primary indicators of the strategic choices caregivers are making in the interest of children's health is that despite an emphasis on symptom management, there is a distinct preference for a biomedical approach when treating HIV.

## SEKHOOA MEDICINE, SESOTHO MEDICINE

One final binary that Basotho negotiate as they encounter illness involves treatment-seeking strategies. Approaches to treatment by biomedical doctors (*ngaka ea Sekhooa*) and Sesotho doctors (*ngaka ea Sesotho*) are drastically different and are based on fundamentally divergent explanatory models and assumptions about the body. However, these approaches are not entirely at odds. Since biomedical treatments have become available and affordable, many sub-Saharan Africans have combined biomedical and indigenous healing practices in selective ways based on their efficacy and their compatibility within a local understanding of disease etiology (Janzen 1981; Cocks and Dold 2000; Kleinman 1980). As Janzen (1981) found among the Kongo of what was then called Zaire, indigenous healers were quick to recognize where biomedical approaches were more effective than indigenous medicines and adjusted their treatment practices accordingly. However, these same healers were also aware of the limitations of biomedical approaches, in particular their inability to address local causes and symptoms of illness, such as witchcraft, pollution, anger, and vulnerability (Janzen 1981). Similarly, Langwick demonstrates how healers in Tanzania blur the boundaries between "science and nonscience" (2011, 7). She puts the current treatment-seeking behaviors of Tanzanians and the practices of local healers in historical and political-economic context by examining the ways that "colonization, missionization, postcolonial state building, international development, and transnational capitalism have shaped the practices known as healing" (Langwick 2011, 7). Following a similar approach, many Basotho combine self-made herbal remedies, indigenous healing practices, prayer, and biomedicine when seeking treatment for a health problem for themselves or the children in their care. As with the seemingly contradictory explanations for illness and the management of symptoms, Basotho view the availability of treatment options as an opportunity to draw on multiple resources in different contexts. As Henderson (2011) also found in rural KwaZulu-Natal, indigenous and biomedical approaches to healing are different, yet they are intertwined, and people must find novel ways to integrate them. In Mokhotlong, patients' and caregivers' treatment-seeking strategies reflect the view of people not merely as biomedicalized bodies but as socially embedded persons.

While many Basotho seek biomedical care, Sesotho medicine remains popular in rural Mokhotlong. The markets and taxi stands in the capital of Maseru and the main roads through every district camptown are lined with the booths of Sesotho doctors, displaying a wide range of herbs, extracts, and roots. Many booths have small private enclosures made of sheets or tarps, where Sesotho doctors can perform consultations and procedures, although they also make house calls. Sesotho doctors like 'M'e Malelang and Ntate Leseko do not use blood tests, X-rays, or other diagnostics that may indicate the underlying cause of illness. Instead, they rely largely on symptoms—both physical and social—to detect illness. Once those symptoms disappear, it is often assumed that the illness is gone, and well-being has been restored. The continued existence of indigenous healers is evidence of the economic viability of the profession and the cultural need that many people have for treatment that extends beyond the biomedical (Langwick 2011). However, many Basotho have mixed feelings about Sesotho medicine. While some view Sesotho doctors as useful for certain things, others dismiss them as dishonest and ineffectual. Those who seek treatment for HIV from Sesotho doctors are in the minority, as the increased availability of free ART and the visible improvement it has made in many patients' lives have encouraged a biomedical approach. Many people in Mokhotlong have adapted to the availability of new pharmaceutical drugs by combining indigenous and biomedical approaches in a way that balances their desire to improve their physical well-being while working within the constraints of their social networks and understandings of disease.

Often Basotho people's treatment-seeking behavior is guided by whether the medical issue is considered a "modern" illness or a "Sesotho" illness, a distinction that manifests itself symptomatically on the body. Sesotho doctors and patients identify Sesotho illnesses by clusters of symptoms commonly attributed to specific local disease categories. In contrast, illnesses perceived to be foreign-born, such as HIV and TB, are often more difficult to pinpoint symptomatically and necessitate listening or looking inside the body—a skill believed to be mastered by biomedical doctors. Despite the often unpleasant side effects of antiretroviral drugs, Basotho generally seek biomedical treatments for HIV. There also appears to be a more general shift away from indigenous healing to biomedical approaches as non-Sesotho illnesses such as HIV and TB become more prevalent and as young, educated Basotho look to align themselves with signs of modernity and distance themselves from traditional practices, which are considered *Sotho-sotho-sotho* (very Sesotho). While some people do not seek care from practitioners of Sesotho medicine, everyday life for rural Basotho is still saturated with home remedies, local understandings of bodies, and conceptions of disease etiology that extend beyond germ theory. A biocultural approach to understanding health and healing in Mokhotlong is essential, even for those who do not consider themselves *Sotho-sotho-sotho*.

In Lesotho, biomedical doctors at the hospitals and clinics are called *ngaka ea Sekhooa*, which translates literally into "English doctors," despite the fact that few of them speak English as a first language. The majority are African (mostly from Zimbabwe, Kenya, and the Democratic Republic of the Congo), although there are also some Americans, Cubans, and Europeans from various countries. Here the word *Sekhooa* simultaneously connotes "English," "foreign," and "modern" and corresponds to a set of ideas about the pathology of illness, the body, and treatments associated with biomedicine. In contrast, indigenous healers in Lesotho are called *ngaka ea Sesotho* (Sesotho doctors), with the word *Sesotho* referring to cultural norms of which the Sesotho language is a part. Yet even as there is a shift in favor of biomedical treatments over indigenous ones, particularly when treating HIV, Basotho de-emphasize biomedical knowledge. As I discovered, people are interested in receiving effective treatments, but they are slow to acknowledge the underlying implications of the transmission and etiology of disease, particularly if it threatens their social relationships.

In general, I witnessed treatment-seeking behavior that favored biomedical intervention but strategically sought out care from Sesotho doctors and indigenous remedies for certain types of ailments—mostly those that Basotho viewed as being distinctly Sesotho illnesses. Medical and epistemological tensions do exist between the two approaches. Patients are often specifically told (by both types of practitioners and by NGOs like MCS) not to mix prescribed pharmaceutical drugs and Sesotho medicines. However, they reconcile these approaches by viewing them as serving distinctly different functions. One young HIV-positive mother, 'M'e Mamohato, told me that when she or her children were sick she would go to both kinds of doctors. She advised me, "If you are sick, because you will not know what you are suffering from, it is better if you can go to both doctors so that they can see your illness. But sometimes if you go to one doctor, it's true that they will give you pills, and you will say you are OK. And when it comes back again, it comes worse than before." 'M'e Mamohato implied that the two different types of doctors might arrive at different diagnoses. Knowledge about both possible ailments allowed her to make a more informed decision about her treatment options. For some types of ailments, 'M'e Mamohato told me that she would first try to make a medicine at home or go to a Sesotho doctor but still thought it best to visit the clinic as well. She advised, "There are diseases that when you have taken Sesotho medicines and when they get better, you should go to the doctor. Even if you are better 100 percent, but you should go to the doctor." However, she told me that illnesses derived from witchcraft were best handled by Sesotho doctors. She explained, "Like now, you see I'm able to see. And the next day, I'm not able to see at all. Like the diseases that are brought by the witches, they are made by people." Still unclear about which ailments were likely to be caused by witchcraft, I asked her how she would know if something needed the attention of a Sesotho doctor. "*Ache!*" she exclaimed, exasperated, "sometimes I might think that I was still living well yesterday, but today,

I have knee pain, and let me go to the Sesotho doctor first. I will go to the *Sekhooa* [biomedical] doctor later." In other words, if an illness or ailment came on unexpectedly, witchcraft was a distinct possibility. Although many Sesotho and biomedical doctors see each other's treatments as contradictory, 'M'e Mamohato viewed them as a network of resources from which to draw strategically.

Other illnesses frequently treated by Sesotho doctors are considered "Sesotho illnesses" and do not have English translations. They are local illnesses characterized by distinct and culturally recognized symptom clusters. For example, *letsoejane* is a sickness common in children, characterized by a fever, heavy breathing, fatigue, and sharp pain. *Nonyana* (bird) is found in babies and looks like a diaper rash but can appear on the back of the head and body. Basotho attribute *nonyana* to mothers who did not drink *pitsa* (a medicine made out of the roots of the *qobo* plant) during childbirth. *Kokoana* is an illness that causes redness in the nose, mouth, and other bodily orifices and is thought to be caused by insects. Similar characterizations of local illnesses exist in many other places in the region, such as in Botswana, where a "complex disease category" often incorporates the symptoms of many common illnesses, such as polio, meningitis, and malnutrition (Klaits 2010). Basotho used to attribute the symptoms of AIDS to a local illness called *mokaola*, until it became more widely diagnosable and treatable (see chapter 3). When Basotho present with symptoms of such "Sesotho illnesses," they are more likely to seek a home remedy or help from a Sesotho doctor. 'M'e Malefu, the village health worker, took her sick daughter to both types of doctors during her illness (which she says was not HIV). When she described the illness to the Sesotho doctor, he told her that the symptoms of abdomen pain, chest pain, and vomiting were "things for Basotho." Unfortunately, neither type of doctor was able to treat her daughter's illness, and she died undiagnosed.

However, a pluralistic approach to treatment is not universal. There appears to be a general move away from Sesotho medicine, particularly among younger Basotho but among elderly caregivers as well. Some of the young and old caregivers I spoke with never sought treatment from Sesotho doctors for themselves or the children in their care, while others were outwardly scornful. For example, 18-year-old 'M'e Masenate said, "I'm afraid of Sesotho doctors. I go to the *Sekhooa* [biomedical] doctors." Others, such as elderly 'M'e Masekha, were harsher in their opinions. She said that she never visited Sesotho doctors: "Sesotho doctors are liars. That's why I don't go to Sesotho doctors." 'M'e Maliapeng, a woman in her mid-40s, agreed, "*Hae*! The Sesotho doctors are lying. People are just paying them, and they are always saying they are going to cure them, yet they are not." Significantly, 'M'e Maliapeng's health had markedly improved after starting ART, so her faith in a biomedical approach was bolstered at that time. 'M'e Matsepiso, who saw her young son Tsepiso recover from near death after receiving TB and HIV treatment, explained that there is a shift toward a bio-medical approach because the illnesses that are now killing Basotho are not Sesotho illnesses. She said, "I don't think there is a cure from the Sesotho doctors. There is only a cure from the *Sekhooa* [biomedical] doctors. It's better if you take them to the clinic. Sesotho is not helpful now." The unspoken implica tion here is that Sesotho medicine may have been useful in the past, but it has become irrelevant as "modern" illnesses increasingly affect Basotho.

In tandem with a declining faith in Sesotho doctors—particularly for treating illnesses perceived as "modern"—comes an attitude toward biomedical doctors that can range from cautious deference to blind confidence. When I was visiting a child living with HIV, her caregiver told me about a new medication she was giving the girl. When pressed, the caregiver did not know what the medication was—whether an ARV or painkiller or vitamin. It turned out to be a common antibiotic, which the girl had been taking previously, just in different packaging. The caregiver was administering the girl's medication as directed based on a deep and unquestioning faith in the biomedical doctor, a faith that had grown in part out of the transformative effect ARVs had on the child's health. Yet interactions between biomedical doctors and nurses and their patients are invariably fraught. Health care providers are chronically overworked, and they lack the resources to provide patients with optimal treatment and care. Furthermore, language barri-ers and biomedical cultural practices in clinical spaces create a context for inter-actions that are power-laden and coercive, and patient knowledge and autonomy rank very low in the hierarchy of concerns.

Interactions between patients and health care providers at the clinics and hospitals often involve very little conversation, with patients rarely asking questions. Patients frequently travel long distances to the hospital or clinic and wait hours to see the doctor but often are not informed of their diagnoses. The doctor merely writes their symptoms and prescriptions in their health booklet (*bukana*), then ushers them into the hallway to wait in another long queue for the pharmacy.[5] Even so, most patients expressed great faith in the recommen-dations of biomedical doctors. This combination of faith and deference was on display when 'M'e Matau told me about people's reactions to her grand-son's recovery after being near death: "We are afraid of *makhooa* [biomedical doctors] if this child is old. They are saying that, and they said they know big things. They didn't think this child would survive." The power of *makhooa* to cure such a sick child so that he could grow "old" reinforces the perceived potency of biomedical doctors and their treatments while at the same time referencing the powerful magic feared and employed by witches and Sesotho doctors.

For patients like 'M'e Masello, such confidence emerged from past positive experiences with biomedical doctors and medications. When I asked 'M'e

Masello—whose chronic asthma had been correctly diagnosed and treated by biomedical doctors—if they ever made a mistake, she responded, "They are always right. Let me tell you from the beginning, beginning, beginning. This thing that I'm suffering from [asthma], they said, every winter I should go to the place where it's warm. This thing doesn't like the cold at all. And I once went to the lowlands, and when I was there, ah ah, [the asthma] wasn't there." Based on her symptoms, she and her family members were convinced that she had TB, yet her chest X-rays repeatedly came back negative. Upon being correctly diagnosed with asthma and experiencing improved health because of relocation and a prescription inhaler, she expressed approval at the biomedical doctors' ability to look beyond the symptoms to make a correct diagnosis.

Confidence also stemmed from the tools of the biomedical doctors' trade, which were perceived as being authoritative and infallible. Several people expressed a preference for biomedical doctors because, unlike the Sesotho doctors, they listened to your body using a stethoscope, a tool that Wendland (2010) notes is also revered by Malawian patients and medical students. 'M'e Malefu echoed the sentiments of others who used Sesotho medicines only for externally identifiable illnesses: "Every illness in the body needs the *Sekhooa* [biomedical] doctor because Basotho don't know the illnesses of the body. And *makhooa* [foreigners or white people] know because they put metal and listen." In 'M'e Malefu's eyes, the biomedical doctors' ability to understand illnesses whose symptoms were hidden or internal made them better suited to treat modern illnesses such as HIV. Many patients, similar to 'M'e Mapoloko, also saw the pen as an authoritative tool: "I think they are correct because they are writing them in the [health] booklet."

Coming from a medical tradition that values patient autonomy and encourages dialogue, I was struck by the lack of communication between biomedical doctors and their patients and by how little this seemed to bother the patients. I was visiting 'M'e Mamorena, Hopolang's paternal great-grandmother, who had recently returned from seeing a doctor at the hospital for stomach pain. She had been given medication but no diagnosis. I asked her if she wanted to know what was going on.

'M'E MAMORENA: Yes, I wanted to know, but he did not tell me.
ELLEN: Why didn't you ask?
'M'E MAMORENA: I asked, but he ignored me. I was asking him, "Why don't you tell me what is going wrong with my stomach?" And he was laughing at me.
ELLEN: So were you angry with the doctor?
'M'E MAMORENA: Ah ah [no], I wasn't angry. We were laughing.
ELLEN: Why not?

'M'E MAMORENA: It's because I have seen that the *Sekhooa* [biomedical] doctor does not explain. And they will not tell you like Sesotho doctors. . . . They don't tell people. I have seen that. They just cure people.

ELLEN: Do you think doctors can make mistakes or be wrong?

'M'E MAMORENA: Ah ah [no]. They can't be wrong.

ELLEN: What do you like about going to the hospital?

'M'E MAMORENA: I want them to listen to me, to use the metal [stethoscope]. Even if they won't tell me, but I want them to put it there [pointing to chest]. To listen that here's like this, here's like this. Even if they don't tell me.

Again, the biomedical doctor's ability to listen inside the body was a source of comfort for 'M'e Mamorena and a source of authority enabled by superior technology.

Many patients also noted being rushed while receiving medical care at the hospitals and clinics. 'M'e Maliapeng told me that she had not yet encountered anyone who communicated well with her while at the doctor. I asked her if she had ever inquired about it, and she said, "*Kannete* [I swear], I haven't asked them because sometimes after you tell them your problem, they just say you should leave quickly. After they have written all the things that you need, they say, 'Go out, go, go, go.'" Although she seemed slightly more annoyed than 'M'e Mamorena, she said that it did not alter her treatment-seeking behaviors because the doctors listened to your problem and could "solve it." Eighteen-year-old 'M'e Masenate also believed that biomedical doctors never made mistakes—in fact, she claimed that if there was an error, it was likely the fault of the pharmacist, who provided the wrong medications. However, unlike 'M'e Maliapeng, she did not think the doctors even listened to patients. I asked her why she did not ask the doctor more questions, and she laughed while describing the following rushed scene: "They are always in a hurry. The doctor will be touching you and saying, 'What are you suffering from? Where is it painful?' while he is writing. And then he will ring the bell for the other patient to come in. Fast. They will say, 'Go out, 'M'e, go out.' And the other patient will be coming in. And you are supposed to go out."

'M'e Malefu, a village health worker and caregiver for two teenaged orphan girls, had a similar experience as 'M'e Maliapeng, but in a rare expression of dissatisfaction, she was not as forgiving of the poor treatment she received at the hospital.

ELLEN: Do you think they should be telling you more without you having to ask the questions?

'M'E MALEFU: Yes, because I am expecting them to tell because I have gone there to tell me what is going on so that I can care for myself.

ELLEN: Have the doctors ever made mistakes?

'M'E MALEFU: Yes, when I enter the door, before I explain, you will see them writing in the book, and when I explain to tell them that I have problems here and here, they will say, "Yes, I have already written that," and I'm always complaining that they have not worked for me.

ELLEN: So you think the doctor is just guessing?

'M'E MALEFU: Yes, I just think when looking at people's faces, they just guess. They just think this person is suffering from this and this and this. I just think they write the wrong things because I have not explained what I'm suffering from.

'M'e Malefu is the same village health worker who told me that she did not always finish her medications when symptoms lessened. She also mentioned that information could help her better care for herself. Perhaps her faith in biomedical authority was weakened by increased exposure to biomedical practices and information through her village health-worker trainings. Those without the benefit of knowledge and training may see no advantage to improved communication with health care providers, despite awareness about the pitfalls of the current medical system.

I witnessed a number of failings on the part of medical staff during my time in Lesotho, some of which directly resulted in loss of life for both adults and children. And yet these medical errors need to be contextualized in the face of extreme personnel shortages and other structural imbalances. Rushed doctor-patient interactions are the result of overworked health professionals and limited diagnostic tools and medical supplies. These structural impediments to optimal health care make many Basotho's acceptance of biomedical authority worrisome, as doctors are prone to errors and misdiagnoses because of the severe shortage of human resources. While I lived in Mokhotlong, there was a steady flow of doctors through the hospital: mostly foreigners. Lesotho does not have a medical school, but it does train nurses, and many Kenyan nurses also work in the country. Maintaining a sufficient number of doctors at the hospital was a challenge. At one point, shortly after I left Lesotho in 2009, a mini-exodus took place: several Cuban doctors completed their contracts; two doctors, including the district medical officer, left to take positions elsewhere in the country; and two others left to take better-paying positions in Botswana. This left only one Congolese doctor—Dr. Mike—at the public hospital. Dr. Mike was the sole doctor on call, 24 hours a day, servicing a district population of 100,000 people. For nearly a month, he was the only person who could do rounds, work the outpatient clinic, or perform emergency surgeries such as C-sections. Even though the countrywide ratio of doctors to patients is 1.15:1,000 (WHO 2006), this ratio is lower—and far more variable—in the rural mountain districts.

HIV necessitates biomedical intervention. From a public health and medical perspective, it is essential that Basotho continue to undergo HIV testing and adhere to antiretroviral treatments. During my fieldwork, I spent much time at the Lerato Center, where ART patients receive treatment at the Mokhotlong Hospital. Despite ongoing stigma surrounding HIV, I was impressed by people's willingness to sit and wait in the open with the other patients, thereby acknowledging their HIV status or the status of the children in their care. As one caregiver told me, "Ah ah, *kannete*, I wasn't afraid. To that door, I went straight to it!" Many ART patients noted that even though they were likely to run into someone they knew, all the other patients were also living with HIV, so there was a reduced fear of being stigmatized. Their willingness to seek treatment at Lerato was not only a sign of stigma reduction—it also pointed to Basotho's strategic use of treatment options to manage care. Caregivers have learned that they can provide better care for an HIV-positive child by denying knowledge about disease transmission while still adhering to a biomedical treatment regimen. At the Lerato Center, the potential for social stigmatization was secondary to the importance of receiving ART.

Basotho seeking biomedical treatment for HIV do not do so to the exclusion of indigenous healing practices. Several South African studies have noted the selective and continued use of indigenous medicines among HIV patients, including those on ART (Peltzer et al. 2008; Babb et al. 2007; Moshabela et al. 2011). However, some of these same studies found that after ART was established, the use of indigenous medicines declined sharply (Peltzer et al. 2010; Moshabela et al. 2011). In the absence of effective treatment, people tend to seek nonbiomedical explanations for infirmity. Haitians attributed tuberculosis to witchcraft until treatments became widely available, after which airborne infection was acknowledged as the cause (Farmer 2004). My own experience confirms that while many HIV patients and caregivers continued to seek care from Sesotho doctors for some ailments, they typically did not visit indigenous healers when they were seeking treatment for issues they perceived as directly related to HIV. This was particularly pronounced once ART was well established, and the benefits of treatment became evident while the side effects lessened. Of course, disentangling particular symptoms and bodily responses as related to HIV or some other ailment is not nearly so straightforward. Even those caregivers who eschewed Sesotho doctors frequently kept a variety of Sesotho medicines on hand to deal with the common aches and pains, cuts, sores, and emotional troubles that living with HIV can bring. My affiliation with MCS—which promotes an allopathic approach to treating HIV and insists that caregivers adhere to the children's biomedical treatment regimens—lessened the likelihood that I would witness people using pluralistic treatment strategies for HIV. Yet the vehemence with which some of the caregivers dismissed Sesotho doctors suggests that a move away from indigenous healing methods as a broad healing strategy is currently under way.

Among the poor, choices are constrained by poverty and structural inequality, and the use of indigenous medicines for certain ailments is sometimes the product of unavailable and unaffordable biomedical therapies (Romero-Daza 2002). In Mokhotlong, silent acceptance of what Lock and Kaufert call the "taken-for-granted knowledge" in biomedicine (1998, 6) gives biomedical practitioners power over the bodies of their patients in problematic ways. In a community with low rates of education, particularly among the elderly, this acceptance of authority is pronounced. Health care providers and policy makers need to be particularly careful of the power dynamics and the ways in which they play out in marginalized communities, especially postcolonial and postapartheid communities. However, as Lock (2001) has warned, it is precisely the need for medicalization that increases the likelihood that imbalances of power and political coercion will be obfuscated in the interest of stopping the progress of illness. Yet Lock (1993) points out elsewhere that biomedical practices are also places for agency and defiance. Although Mokhotlong residents may not exercise this agency in their interactions with medical authority, they may do so in the privacy of their homes, as they make choices about their own treatments and care. For example, 'M'e Malefu visited the hospitals and clinics and did not openly challenge the doctors. At home, however, she chose how and when to administer her medication. In many cases of poor adherence, patients disliked the side effects of ARVs and ceased taking them.

The continued, if declining, use of Sesotho doctors indicates the inadequacy of biomedical methods alone to respond to people's physical, emotional, cultural, and spiritual needs. Lock and Kaufert argue that "the claims of medical knowledge to a privileged status depend on the belief, shared by medical professionals and the public alike, that scientific knowledge, being factual, cannot be subjected to epistemological scrutiny" (Lock and Kaufert 1998, 6). Hospitals and clinics discourage their patients from seeking treatment from indigenous healers, yet a collaborative approach that provides community-based services for HIV can be particularly effective in addressing the complex needs of patients. In one pilot study in Lesotho, Sesotho doctors successfully participated in the roll-out of ART, which included promoting testing and prevention as well as monitoring patients (Furin 2011). While medical knowledge does have authority in Mokhotlong, faith in biomedicine is not totalizing and does not preclude a simultaneous faith in indigenous healing or supernatural disease etiologies. Basotho are comfortable with the inherent tensions in their syncretic beliefs. When confronted with the apparent binaries involved in disease and treatment, many Mokhotlong residents take a pluralistic approach. This allows them to selectively engage with a range of choices in order to expand and improve their health outcomes and protect their networks of care. Yet the delicate balance sought by patients seeking biomedicine and indigenous medicine reinforces the ways that culture is constrained and shaped by structural inequalities.

## CONCLUSION: CONTRADICTIONS OR ADAPTATIONS?

When confronted with illness, Basotho strategically present various explanations for illness and treatment-seeking behaviors, based on complex motivational, structural, and temporal factors. They draw from multiple resources and explanatory models in ways that privilege health, kin relationships, and care. Caregivers and patients emphasize a nonbiomedical or religious causality, which helps remove blame regarding modes of transmission, reduces stigma that could threaten networks of care, and protects the memory of loved ones. Yet they demonstrate knowledge about the biomedical causes of illness when it is necessary for access to therapeutic resources. Likewise, although Basotho tend to manage illness by focusing on symptom resolution, they continue to take medications even after symptoms have reduced when they view it as beneficial to health—such as when treating HIV and TB. Finally, they employ pluralistic treatment strategies, drawing on both biomedical and nonbiomedical approaches depending on their assessment of the type of treatment available that would best meet their needs at that moment. The negotiations around these binaries are strategies that expand the resources of communities with many structural disadvantages and that reflect a biosocial approach to health.

Many Mokhotlong residents treat Sesotho illnesses (identified by locally defined symptom clusters) by seeking care from Sesotho doctors. In contrast, illnesses that are viewed as being "modern," foreign, or internal to the body are treated with biomedicine. Sustained HIV- and TB-prevalence rates necessitate increased biomedicalization, so Basotho have become more familiar with a biomedical approach. There also seems to be a tendency, particularly among young Basotho and for those whose lives depend on biomedical treatments (such as ARVs), to turn away from Sesotho medicine altogether. This may be linked to the privileged status AIDS enjoys in the public health sphere in Lesotho and to the free and widely available HIV treatments, including any costs associated with opportunistic infections. In contrast, the costs of Sesotho doctors' fees and medicines have become prohibitive for some patients whose resources are already stretched. Even though Basotho no longer seek the treatments of Sesotho doctors as frequently, continued reliance on symptom management poses problems for HIV care, which often does not present itself symptomatically until a patient's viral load is already very high.

The uptake of biomedical treatments for HIV and AIDS is a key component in stopping the further spread of the pandemic. Antiretroviral treatment reduces a patient's viral load, which in turn reduces the likelihood of transmission to sexual partners or from mother to child. Yet the power dynamic that exists between overworked and underpaid health care workers and patients is one of unquestioned authority, especially during the doctor's visit. These uncontested interactions create challenges as patients and caregivers struggle to understand the fundamental nature of the illness and its treatment. They are therefore often unable to respond when challenges of poverty, geography, or political economy arise. Even as Basotho turn toward biomedical solutions, they turn away from biomedical knowledge that might threaten their social relationships and their networks of care. In an effort to disseminate biomedical knowledge to patients—of HIV or any other disease—there is a need to recognize this tension and to present biomedical knowledge in a way that enhances care without challenging the role of the caregiver. The unquestioned acceptance of biomedical knowledge is problematic because it impairs the ability for caregivers to make decisions and to advocate for children and for themselves. As the following chapter illuminates, the fundamental issues related to illness and treatment presented here shape the ways that Basotho view HIV prevention, testing, and treatment—and therefore, the ways they care for orphans.

# 3 · "LIKE ANY OTHER DISEASE"

## The River of Voices

*I first met Lebo in June of 2007, when he was 19 months old. Back then, he was HIV positive, and later he wasn't.*

*At that time, Lebo lived in a small village off the road from Mokhotlong to Mapholaneng, the same winding road where many years later, my two children and I would make a daredevil run through the mountains to get petrol. There hadn't been a fume in Mokhotlong for weeks, so when a rumor blew through town that a petrol tanker had made its way up to Mapholaneng, I strapped the kids into their car seats and asked myself if perhaps this was a terrible idea. But by that point, the plan had acquired a certain momentum—now or never—and it was this same momentum that carried us all the way to Mapholaneng with the needle buried in red, coasting down long gradual drops into the valley before kicking the car into gear as we climbed. We rollercoaster'd like this for 40 minutes, dropping in and out of neutral, and as we crested the final ridge, a Taylor Swift song came on the radio. It would be wrong to say we didn't feel triumphant.*

*Anyway, it probably was a dumb idea—child endangerment based on rumors and hearsay—although sometimes that's all you've got to go on. Word travels briskly through the mountains, but nuance snags easily on spiky outcroppings, and meaning can get tumbled in the wind.*

\* \* \*

*I knew Lebo long before I knew my own children, though. I loved that boy desperately. It was the first time I'd cared for a child who—as I journaled at the time, during my first visit to MCS (Mokhotlong Children's Services)—"had an invisible countdown until his tiny body gave out." I shudder now at that melodramatic and essentializing sentiment, but that was how I first understood him.*

*It was a particularly confusing sentiment too, because by June 2007, after several months of ART (antiretroviral therapy), Lebo's meds had kicked in, and his lively*

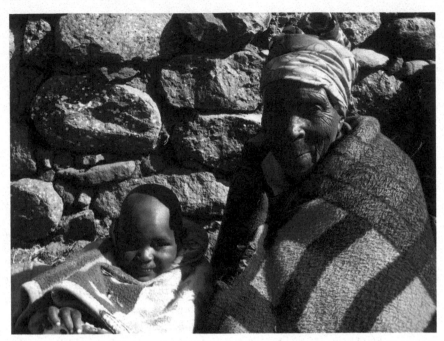

FIGURE 3.1. Lebo and his great-grandmother, 'M'e Masello, sit in front of their home to warm up, Mokhotlong, 2009

*personality had emerged from some immunosuppressed hibernation: Lebo the overca-ffeinated joybot, a fat-cheeked goof forever dressed in a generic red sports jersey. Daily, I steered him away from the smaller and more introverted babies at MCS, who dis-liked his tackle-hugs and the attendant rug burn. At lunchtime, I would spoon mashed banana into his mouth, which he would receive calmly before extruding it through pursed lips while I was readying the next bite. In the afternoons, I would rock him in the toddler seat of a rudimentary swing set that someone had bribed across the South African border. One afternoon, he fell asleep there, flopped forward in sunny repose, before he woke and loudly filled the swing's bucket seat with pea-green diarrhea.*

*Lebo's parents were both dead. His great-grandmother was his primary caregiver, and it was she who had taken him to the hospital after his chronic stomach problems refused to dissipate. From the hospital, he was discharged to MCS. One afternoon, after Lebo had been at MCS for several months, his great-grandmother came to visit him. It was the first time she had been able to make the journey. Nkhono clapped happily and cooed over the boy, thrilled by his obvious weight gain, but Lebo clung to me. He didn't know who she was.*

\* \* \*

Once Lebo's health evened out and once 'M'e Nthabiseng felt convinced that the boy's caregiving situation was stable, Lebo returned to live with his great-grandmother, 'M'e Masello. This was in November of 2007, after he had been at MCS for 11 months. Back then, Lebo was one more sweet boy navigating the complicated realities of HIV, and back then, 'M'e Masello was one more caregiver doing her best to pick out meaning from the confusing swirl of voices—outreach worker, doctor, nurse, well-meaning anthropologist—each voice washing over the others, clamoring to explain what HIV was and what it meant.

As 'M'e Masello took the taxi out of town, she would have passed the lone billboard on the road to Mapholaneng. **ABC**, the sign read in bold letters: **A**bstinence, **B**e faithful, **C**ondomize. This was the government's advice on how to defeat the spread of HIV. But what to make of the people in her village who said that condoms caused HIV, not prevented it? One neighbor had seen with her own eyes—well, not with her own eyes, but the neighbor knew someone who had seen it—how tiny worms lived inside condoms, worms that carried that disease. It could be proved, the neighbor said; she had done it herself—well, not personally, but she knew someone who had—how if you took a condom and boiled it and left it in the sun, you could see those worms crawling out.

The story sounded farfetched, but so many people said it was true. And anyway—how could a husband and wife even use a condom? It was either an accusation of infidelity or a confession of it. 'M'e Masello tried to imagine asking her husband—long dead now; how long had it even been?—to use that khohlopo during sex. The thought alone was ridiculous.

As for the other part, on Sundays, the preacher talked about abstinence—an easy thing to say from the pulpit, but who really behaved like that? The whole thing was too confusing. Everyone knew something different about that disease: the Sekhooa doctors and the Sesotho doctors and the neighbors and the anthropologist and the billboards and the voices on the taxi's radio—a whirlwind of truth and rumor, hearsay and fact.

The only things nkhono could really trust, it seemed, were her own eyes. And all they could see was that Lebo's symptoms were getting better every day he took his medication.

\* \* \*

By January 2009, Ellen and I had returned to Mokhotlong after more than a year in the United States. It was around this time that a glorious and impossible rumor reached us: Lebo was no longer HIV positive. The boy was healthy, people said. It was a miracle—he was no longer even an MCS client. We rolled our eyes. We knew the danger of giving in to hope; we knew how stories traveled through the mountains, how meaning got tumbled in high winds.

But when Ellen visited his village, she found that the impossible was true: Lebo was HIV negative. He had been retested three separate times now, MCS had consulted with several doctors, and it was confirmed. The original test had been a false positive—rare but not unheard of—and the doctors had now taken him off his meds. They wondered aloud if perhaps his bloodwork had gotten mixed-up in the lab, and Lebo's great-grandmother must have wondered if it was even HIV to begin with. In the village, people sometimes said that the disease wasn't real or that it was something the makhooa—the foreigners—had created. Others claimed it was just a different name for Sesotho diseases, kokoana or mokaola or mofetse, these things that Sesotho doctors knew how to cure. Because if it was HIV, how could it be cured? 'M'e Masello knew that much; the village health worker had told her the illness of H was incurable. She had heard people saying similar things on the radio too, those voices calling in to share their stories, people arguing about that disease for the youth. But those voices said crazy things too, like HIV came from having too many abortions, and that couldn't be right, could it?

It didn't matter. The only truth was that her sweet boy was cured. She had seen it with her own eyes.

In the rondavel that day, Ellen and nkhono sat talking. She was telling Ellen stories about the old days, about growing up in the village. 'M'e Masello could laugh about it now, especially on this day of happy news, but she described how the older times were ruled by silence and whispers. She had only learned of sex on the night of her marriage—"If the river had not been full then, I would have run away from that painful thing!" she said. She described how especially with things like sex and pregnancy and childbirth—with matters of kinship—it was secrecy that defined them. Back when she was 15 and newly married, they told her that a woman would go down to the river and find her baby there among the reeds. "Ache!"—she was laughing and shaking her head—"We really believed it then. We were married like that, not knowing anything."

But those were the old ways. Nkhono told Ellen that the children today no longer believe those stories, they laugh at the rumors and myths, and this is a good thing. "Thuto ke bophelo," she said. "Education is life."

Before Ellen left that day, Lebo and his siblings came out to gawp at Ellen's motorcycle. She held them in the saddle of her parked dirt bike, and Lebo and the other kids posed proudly.

'M'e Masello was standing in the doorway of the rondavel. "If you could see inside me," she told Ellen, "you would see how my heart is moving."

* * *

But you know how stories go. This is a story just like any other.

The weather turned cold, and the harvest came, leaving a patchwork of gold and rust across the mountains. People stayed in their rondavels and talked and laughed and worried, circulating old myths and new rumors. Everyone was talking, and when the talk turned to that disease, all the voices overlapped.

After the harvest, Ellen rode out to the village to say hello and found Lebo sick. 'M'e Masello said that he had been complaining about his stomach again and was suffering from chronic diarrhea. She was planning to take him to the hospital the following day. Ellen told 'M'e Masello to come visit MCS after they were done there—all the staff would want to see that sweet boy again.

At the hospital the next day, the doctors gave Lebo something for his diarrhea—told nkhono that it would reduce symptoms—then sent them on their way.

When they arrived at MCS, 'M'e Nthabiseng took one look at Lebo and walked him into her office. She retested him on the spot.

By this point, Lebo had been off his meds for more than a year.

* * *

How to explain something like this? Ellen tried, but hers was just one more voice in a river of voices—the Sekhooa doctors and Sesotho doctors, the billboards and the pastors, the talk-radio call-ins and the people in the village—everyone with something to say about HIV and all the voices washing together.

Ellen was sitting with 'M'e Masello in her rondavel. This was a month after the terrible result had come back that day in 'M'e Nthabiseng's office. Lebo was back on ARVs (antiretroviral drugs) now.

"I was so surprised when they first said it had gone away," nkhono told Ellen. "How has it gone and yet they say there is no cure? I was just asking myself and answering myself. They were the ones who said it has gone; they were the ones who stopped Lebo's services. And I didn't say anything because I didn't know anything." 'M'e Masello had wanted so badly to believe the Sekhooa doctors. How had they gotten it so wrong?

'M'e Masello shook her head, and Ellen said—no, she didn't say anything. Sometimes the only thing to do is listen.

"And now they've told me he is positive again," nkhono continued. "I was so angry. I thought they were playing with me. They were the ones who stopped his services." She launched into a coughing fit, hacking and wheezing in the rondavel.

After a while, Ellen asked if 'M'e Masello wanted to know what had happened.

"Yes," she said, still trying to settle her breathing. "If it is possible, I want to know."

Ellen explained that when Lebo had initially tested HIV positive, back when he first came to MCS, it was an accurate result. The standard practice is to retest several times, though—at six weeks out and again at a few months out—since small children can carry antibodies from their mothers, which will sometimes produce false positives in healthy children. But by the time Lebo was retested at six months out, his body had responded so well to ART that the test was no longer able to detect the disease. The several tests that followed all seemed to confirm that he was HIV-free, and so the doctors concluded that the very first test had been a false positive. But the disease had always been there, lurking at times below detectable levels, a devastating anomaly.

They sat there in silence for a while. "It was no one's fault, nkhono," Ellen said. "Not the doctors at the hospital or the staff at MCS. Sometimes it just happens."

She wondered if this was true.

\* \* \*

And so we are back where we began, with a sweet boy named Lebo who is HIV positive, now for the second time. By late 2009, he is thriving again—the meds are doing their job—and 'M'e Masello is happy with his progress. "He is becoming fat compared to before," she told Ellen. "He took a long time vomiting and having diarrhea and not eating anything, but now he is no longer tired like he was; he's playing and growing strong."

She stopped for a moment, wheezing again.

"If I was a dog," she said, "I would be wagging my tail. Kannete, I'm happy."

But surely it is not an uncomplicated happiness, for 'M'e Masello faces the conundrum of knowing that Lebo's confirmed HIV-positive status has also allowed the family to receive food packages from MCS—their food security now directly tied to Lebo's disease.

And if she is happy, it is a happiness she keeps mostly to herself. She doesn't discuss Lebo's disease or health with anyone in the village, she says. The nurses at the rural clinic told her not to talk about it. So silence reigns again, a return to the old ways, and the whispers and rumors swirl around the edges.

\* \* \*

Ellen and I kept up with Lebo as best we could over the years. We saw him again in 2013, but by that point, 'M'e Masello had died. She knew the end was coming but had left the arrangements for his care to be decided by family members at her funeral. When we saw him, Lebo was living with relatives in another village.

In the rondavel that day, he was quiet—understandably circumspect in the presence of these strange makhooa visitors, following us around the room with wide eyes—but he looked healthy, a lean seven-year-old. His new caregivers said that they were doing their best with his medications. It was complicated at first, they said, but over time, they had become accustomed to the routine.

In 2015, we returned to Mokhotlong again, but this time, we weren't able to visit Lebo. He would have been almost 10 years old then.

Strange—to remember that sweet sturdy goof I held in my arms so many years before. People told us that Lebo was doing well, still healthy, with good adherence to his meds. He must have been in school by then, unless he was already working as a herd boy. Word reached us that his relatives were managing—it was always difficult to take on another hungry child—but they were getting by. At least, that's what people said.

That was the year I coasted with my children through the mountains in a car with no petrol, thinking of Lebo as we passed his old home, rising and falling, hoping all the way that the story we'd heard was true.

-WM-

\* \* \*

## BIOMEDICAL PRIMACY

Lebo's experience with HIV was highly unusual. While inaccurate HIV tests do sometimes occur (see, for example, Sakarovich et al. 2007), I never encountered a situation like Lebo's, with multiple testing and retesting errors. Yet misinformation about HIV, confusion about the accuracy of varying sources of information, and a perception that recommendations for HIV prevention and treatment are constantly in flux are common epistemological challenges for Mokhotlong residents. This type of uncertainty is expected by patients navigating AIDS in Lesotho. And while 'M'e Masello's reluctance to discuss Lebo's status is evidence of ongoing stigma, it is also the result of a general sense of privacy that Basotho have about bodily afflictions, which makes community education challenging. Lebo's story also highlights the role that chance encounters play in the outcomes of children and families in this environment. If I had not run into Lebo at the hospital that day, he may have gone undiagnosed even longer, lessening the chance that treatment would be successful. Given that his CD4 (cluster of differentiation 4) percentage was 13—very low for a child—he likely did not have much time to spare, although his trials over the years had proven him resilient.

Historically, anthropologists comparing ethnomedical systems used cultural relativism as a methodological tool to explore the local social and cultural beliefs and practices surrounding different approaches to health and healing. Following a critical turn in the 1970s and 1980s, medical anthropologists increasingly recognized that any examination of health and healing that did not consider its relationship to global political-economic structures was of little use (Singer 1989). In a time of unfathomable medical progress, residents of Mokhotlong had to contend with many of the pitfalls of health care provision in the Global South: medical technologies that were decades old, funding bodies that poured money into vertical health initiatives (like that for HIV) without strengthening health systems, and leaders who ignored the severity of global health problems unless it was politically expedient to attend to them.

James Pfeiffer and Mark Nichter have called on medical anthropologists to use their ethnographic skills, their reliance on multiple ways of knowing, and their local community-based expertise to bring a critical lens to the unequal distribution of disease in order to "document and contextualize the effectiveness of health services as they impact people's lives" (2008, 412). In Mokhotlong, this type of critical approach is essential for a number of reasons. First, the political-economic context in which HIV has flourished in southern Africa has left many people vulnerable, without the necessary treatment, education, and social supports to combat the disease. Second, the history of public health messages, misinformation, and fatal missteps by political leaders, particularly in neighboring South Africa, set the stage for an epidemic of disastrous proportions throughout the region. And third, in this case, the health knowledge and beliefs of Mokhotlong residents and caregivers are a matter of life and death—only ARVs can extend lives and prevent the transmission of HIV from mother to child. Yet medical technologies in Lesotho are still decades behind costly treatments widely used in the Global North. If we are to strive for health equity, then in this context, providing access to biomedical treatments and reliable health education is the only way to move forward. This can—and should—work in concert with local ways of knowing and healing. However, when assessing rural Basotho's access to knowledge and technologies that will help them live, I do not give equal weight to varying beliefs about ways of preventing and treating HIV.

This work assumes and demonstrates that when it comes to HIV, people generally desire access to the best biomedical treatments available, in addition to indigenous healing practices. The tendency of governments, pharmaceutical companies, and global systems to uphold unequal access to ARVs as merely "cost effective" is highly problematic, and structural inequalities make survival even more difficult in this context. Because of this, I do not shy away from seemingly unanthropological terms such as *biomedical facts, misinformation, accuracy,* and *misconceptions*: in this case, sorting out actual modes of transmission, effective methods of prevention, and proper adherence to treatment is vital. Yet critical medical anthropology takes culture seriously by looking at how structural violence leads to unequal access to care, how cultural beliefs and practices shape people's responses to the information that is available to them, and how people continue to act in ways that protect their social networks whether or not this undermines good health.

In this chapter, I address how AIDS education is pervasive yet inconsistent, resulting in significant gaps in knowledge among the people of Mokhotlong. I then examine how multiple competing sources of information translate into rural Basotho's knowledge about the illness and its impact on the body, once again with a focus on symptom management. Although the widespread availability and visible success of antiretroviral treatments have increased the credibility of the biomedical response to HIV/AIDS, misinformation and misconceptions about the disease continue to impact Basotho's responses to prevention and treatment. These are further complicated by caregivers' attempts to discuss HIV in ways that protect their social networks and familial relationships. I also explore the generational gap in knowledge that exists between young people and the elderly. Although grandparents in Lesotho have not suffered from HIV with nearly the same frequency as their children and grandchildren, grandmothers in particular are largely responsible for the care of HIV-infected orphans; therefore, reducing the HIV knowledge gap among the elderly is essential.

I then delve into Basotho's perceptions and reactions toward prevention, testing, and treatment efforts—the three primary areas of intervention for HIV/AIDS. I describe the culturally specific challenges that exist in these areas of AIDS intervention while attending to ways in which they intersect with gender dynamics, poverty, malnutrition, and geographic realities. I explore such issues as condom use, mother-to-child transmission of HIV, trends in HIV testing, barriers to treatment adherence, and people's responses to the side effects of antiretroviral drugs. The evidence presented here points simultaneously to a decrease in AIDS-related stigma and to its persistence despite significant gains. Ultimately, this close exploration of Basotho's encounters with HIV on multiple levels helps illuminate how HIV is locally understood both as a disease with foreign origins that necessitates biomedical intervention and as a social disease that impacts kin relations.

In this book, I emphasize the importance of sociality and demonstrate the many ways that Basotho privilege kinship and caregiving relationships. Although my primary focus is orphan care and relationships between kin, the current crisis in caregiving is greatly affected by the scale and longevity of the AIDS pandemic and the specific ways it has played out in communities. Local responses to AIDS interventions impact orphans and orphan care because adult behavior affects both the health of caregivers and the health of the children in their care. In the previous chapters, I presented a historicized and contextualized microlevel view of the everyday interactions and negotiations Basotho make with regard to social organization, patterns of household configuration, and beliefs and choices regarding health. These social patterns come to bear on the specific interactions Basotho have with HIV/AIDS information and their experiences with prevention and treatment initiatives. It is at the point where patterns of social organization and practices of care intersect with the realities of living and coping with HIV that the idea of AIDS as a kinship disease comes to life. HIV is not a disease that exists in its own realm and maps onto bodies and populations. The scale of the pandemic in Lesotho means that the disease does not merely *interact* with local environments, but rather, it plays a fundamental role in shaping them. Mokhotlong residents—both consciously and subconsciously—consider the physical and social ramifications of their beliefs and choices when seeking HIV treatment and when caring for loved ones. Their navigation of this is deeply constrained by structural inequalities such as poverty and poor health services, resulting in suboptimal medical treatments. HIV does not merely influence different aspects of social and family life in a haphazard or linear way. Rather, a dialectic relationship exists between HIV and kinship, where Basotho's beliefs and decision-making regarding HIV treatment and care are the result of constant feedback and interactions between structural, biomedical, and cultural aspects of the disease at every level.

The findings presented in this chapter are at once hopeful and discouraging, creating both clarity and confusion. Health and social responses to HIV are improving, as is knowledge about the disease and access to treatment and care. Yet notwithstanding the widespread use of ARVs, HIV transmission rates have not abated as quickly as expected. People are living longer with HIV, yet children are still dying undiagnosed. As Kenworthy and her colleagues (2017) note, the disease marches on even as global interest in it wanes, taking much-needed global funding with it. The stark juxtaposition of rural life and constantly changing medical protocols highlights the complexity and dynamic tension of HIV/AIDS in Mokhotlong, defying simple summary. If anything, the lesson to be learned here is this: the factors impacting children and families are not easily generalizable. Yet understanding them can help improve HIV interventions and strengthen the assertion that AIDS is a kinship disease.

## AIDS (MIS)EDUCATION

The overview of Mokhotlong residents' perceptions of illness and their treatment-seeking behaviors (see chapter 2) helps put the following discussion about HIV/AIDS knowledge, beliefs, and responses to intervention into perspective. Information flow, opinions, and knowledge about HIV vary widely across the population and along lines of age, education, health, and eligibility for services and stem from multiple sources. The information is translated into multiple, sometimes contradictory, understandings of the physical impact HIV has on the body. Basic knowledge about HIV/AIDS in Mokhotlong is pervasive—I met only one very old blind woman who claimed that she knew nothing about it (though she admitted to hearing people talk about it). Yet my interlocutors' knowledge about HIV was inconsistent; so too was their willingness to discuss it openly. Methods of knowledge dissemination that could capitalize on the socially embedded nature of HIV were not being utilized to their fullest potential.

MCS's managing director, 'M'e Nthabiseng, outlined for me her perspective on how information flows in rural communities and how multiple competing sources of information can cause confusion and impede behavior change:

People who at least have gone to school or have access to reading material on HIV . . . even though they don't change their behavior, they still believe there is HIV, based on what information they get and see. But people in the village who really don't have access to a lot of information, they depend on word of mouth, which can change from person to person. And also, HIV as it is, it's complicated because of the information and the way it changes from time to time . . . so I think people are kind of confused, and that leads to them thinking there's no HIV. You know. So within that confusion, they still don't change anything. For them it's one of those sicknesses that maybe there's a cure, maybe there's no cure—that kind of thing.

At the time of this conversation, in 2009, I had noticed considerable changes in attitudes and behaviors around HIV in the few years that I had been working with caregivers in Mokhotlong. Surprised by this pessimistic view, I asked 'M'e Nthabiseng, "So you don't think there have been any changes in the rural areas?" She surmised that change was less apparent the farther you got from town but then qualified her comment: "The changes are really slow compared to the spread of HIV. But there is change."

AIDS education and knowledge has improved across southern Africa, but considerable gaps still exist. In a study of nine African countries, Glick and Sahn (2007) found that knowledge was lowest among rural Africans and women, and differences in knowledge were, perhaps predictably, more pronounced with disparities in wealth and education. South Africans with "traditional" beliefs about the cause of HIV had higher rates of misinformation about prevention and treatment and were more likely to support social stigmatization of people living with the disease (Kalichman and Simbayi 2004). As Mokhotlong is both rural and poor, with low levels of education beyond primary school, the responses of caregivers examined here correspond to the less informed population stratums in the region.

According to Lesotho's 2014 Demographic and Health Survey, knowledge about the *existence* of HIV/AIDS was nearly universal. This is hardly surprising given that one in four people are infected. Yet only 39 percent of young women and 31 percent of young men had comprehensive knowledge about HIV (Lesotho Ministry of Health 2016). Moreover, acknowledging the existence of HIV is not enough to positively influence prevention and treatment outcomes. As Nicola Bulled illustrates, in Lesotho, the top-down flow of information based on Western logics and controlled by experts is insufficient to make any real dent in improving HIV-prevention strategies, largely because culture is treated cursorily at best. She argues that culture needs to be central to health communication strategies and to include the voices and perspectives of the recipients of such information (Bulled 2014). Like Bulled, I observed the inconsistent flow and uptake of health information. Knowledge about HIV was highly variable from person to person, and a single patient's account could shift from one visit to the next. This stems from the plurality of competing messages about HIV/AIDS and the multiple pathways on which knowledge and education about the disease travel. It also stems from the different ways that such knowledge affects people's lives at different times. Information that is likely to affect a loved one positively—information that removes blame, for instance, or information that gives a caregiver hope—is more likely to be seen as credible. Furthermore, there are "official" sources of information such as government-run public health campaigns and unofficial sources such as informal conversations with neighbors. Information from trusted authorities (e.g., community-run support groups, village health workers, chiefs, and pastors) often masks politicized or religious agendas and conveys variable levels of accurate biomedical knowledge. The result is a scattered and varied flow of information that has created considerable confusion about the veracity of AIDS-related information.

Media communication through radio, television, billboards, and posters is commonplace in rural Mokhotlong. Although Basotho living in the outlying villages of Mokhotlong's camptown do not have electricity (and therefore television), most people have occasional access to battery- or solar-powered radio (either their own or a neighbor's). People also listen to the radio during lengthy minibus taxi rides. Media coverage, however, is much lower in the rural areas than in the urban centers. In Mokhotlong, only 14 percent of men and women have weekly access to radio, the most common form of media consumption, compared with more than 40 percent in urban areas (Lesotho Ministry of Health 2016). When rural Basotho encounter these forms of communication, they are inundated with largely positive messages such as those from Lesotho's Know Your Status campaign, which encourages HIV testing. There are call-in shows where people discuss thorny social scenarios stemming from HIV, religious radio broadcasts emphasizing abstinence and faithfulness, and news programs discussing recent advancements in HIV treatment. News reports also chronicle the failures and frustrations of HIV programs and report on political controversies, such as the highly publicized missteps of former South African presidents Thabo Mbeki and Jacob Zuma; even the beloved Nelson Mandela failed to address the emerging AIDS pandemic during his tenure (Fassin 2007; Robins 2008; Mayosi and Benatar 2014).

South Africa's initial response to HIV—characterized by silence, mistrust, fear, and uncertainty—demonstrates the harm that negative press and public misinformation can have on the trajectory of a disease. Most prominently, then-president Thabo Mbeki publicly denied that HIV caused AIDS, a position that researchers estimate cost the lives of 330,000 people and caused 35,000 babies to become HIV infected (Chigwedere et al. 2008). Mbeki's minister of health notoriously earned the moniker Dr. Beetroot, known as she was for encouraging those living with HIV to use natural remedies such as garlic, lemon, and beet-root to cure HIV (Fassin 2007). Jacob Zuma, who succeeded Mbeki as president until he was forced to resign in February of 2018, was accused of rape in 2005 and acquitted the following year. During his highly publicized trial, he claimed that although he had unprotected sex with a woman he knew to be HIV positive, he showered afterward, which he believed reduced the likelihood of transmission (Robins 2008). With such questionable leadership, it is not hard to imagine the confusion ordinary citizens felt about the best ways to prevent and treat HIV, and given South Africa's political and economic prominence, the negative impacts of South Africa's official and unofficial AIDS policies still reverberate across the region.

Reliable biomedical information about HIV often comes from patient interactions with various health care workers, such as doctors, nurses, and voluntary counseling and testing (VCT)[1] personnel, and through the mandatory adherence sessions that HIV-positive adults (and caregivers of HIV-positive children) are required to attend. Basotho also receive information from social workers and NGO employees. However, information is abundant for those "therapeutic citizens" (Nguyen 2005) who are already connected to networks of providers by nature of their roles as "ART patient" or "AIDS orphan"—labels they (or their caregivers) have likely accepted in order to claim eligibility for services. Those who fall outside of these categories are often excluded from their networks of resources, information, and support.

Most Basotho identify as Christian, and church activities and pastors' sermons are important and trusted sources of information about AIDS. Churches are poised to play a significant role as leaders in the response to HIV due to their pervasiveness (Hartwig, Kissioki, and Hartwig 2006; Campbell, Skovdal, and Gibbs 2011), yet many churches in southern Africa were slow to respond to the crisis (Hartwig, Kissioki, and Hartwig 2006; Prince 2009). While churches have helped care for those impacted by HIV, their public response has been highly variable. As Klaits notes of Botswana in the early years of the pandemic, some churches used the pulpit as an opportunity to promote sexual monogamy, some organized care and prevention groups, some publicly denied the existence of AIDS, and some ignored it altogether (Klaits 2010). Many religious leaders and churches have helped by creating "supportive social spaces," challenging stigma, and supporting the care of people living with HIV and orphans (Campbell, Skovdal, and Gibbs 2011). However, churches also have the potential to foster HIV stigma through silence and moralizing messages, by de-emphasizing safe-sex practices, and by reinforcing gender ideologies that disempower women in negotiating for their own health (Hartwig, Kissioki, and Hartwig 2006; Campbell, Skovdal, and Gibbs 2011; Prince 2009; Parsitau 2009).

Given the moral authority of the churches in Mokhotlong, it is essential that religious leaders be thoroughly informed, not only about prevention and treatment but also about communicating positive messages that reduce stigma. 'M'e Malefu, a village health worker and caregiver for two AIDS orphans, said that she had heard her pastor speak many times about HIV. She said that pastors "talk in a positive way to solve this problem." Like many religious leaders, her pastor focused on faithfulness: "They encourage Basotho not to be attracted to other people's partners. Because if it [HIV] wasn't there in your family, and you go to another family, you will get it. And they encourage people to stay at their families—not to go to other people's families." Here the pastor emphasizes the harmful way that HIV spreads through networks of kin. Like 'M'e Malefu's, many pastors are concerned most with faithfulness in marriage. Yet people's religious beliefs and values and their sexual practices are often at odds. Young men and women in Lesotho typically start having sexual intercourse several years before they are married (Lesotho Ministry of Health 2016), and many have multiple concurrent partnerships even after they are married.

Tsepiso's young mother agreed that church leaders were spreading positive messages. She had heard them "encouraging people to know their status, if they realize that all people are dying." Although none of the churchgoing Basotho I spoke with said that they ever heard church leaders discuss HIV in a negative or overtly stigmatizing way, many insisted that it was not a frequent topic of conversation. Some said that they never heard their pastor talk about HIV; others said it was discussed in smaller groups but not in the larger church services. Matseli's grandparents, 'M'e Maliehi and Ntate Kanelo, are devout Catholics. 'M'e Maliehi told me that "even the priests are talking about (HIV) nowadays," telling their parishioners that "you should respect it because it is dangerous." However, they also praised priests for not addressing HIV directly when children were present. I was surprised that 'M'e Maliehi, who was so open with me and with her husband, would value that kind of silence. Ntate Kanelo added approvingly, "Ache, ah ah, the children don't have that mind. Ache, I don't like it." I asked him how children would learn to protect themselves, and he simply said, "When they are older." A culture of silence surrounding sexuality and illness more generally creates barriers for open communication about HIV, hampering AIDS interventions.

Ntate and 'M'e Monatsi, a young husband-and-wife team, are leaders of a local independent Christian church. In conversation with me, they reflected critically on their past reluctance to discuss HIV openly with their congregation, even as they cared for those impacted by AIDS in their homes and communities. Ntate Monatsi had recently returned from a training workshop with the Christian AIDS Bureau of Southern Africa (CABSA), and he was still energized from the transformative experience. Although both husband and wife had been tested and were talking privately with individuals and families about HIV, Ntate

Monatsi felt that they were only now "waking up" to the responsibility they had to spread a Christian approach to HIV—one guided by principles of love, compassion, dignity, and hope. 'M'e Monatsi reflected, "You know, actually taking it into the church, whereby the whole congregation is there and talking about it seriously, it was our first time." Both husband and wife felt that pastors were particularly well situated to bring about positive change because they had "influence" and were "more trustworthy" than other community leaders, like chiefs (an opinion obviously not shared by the chiefs themselves). Ntate Monatsi thoughtfully described the superficial treatment of past AIDS education initiatives in his own church:

> Over and over and over . . . people know if there is an HIV/AIDS workshop, it's OK: talk about sex a little bit, laugh a little bit, eat, and go home. . . . Since the workshops have been run here, nothing has happened in order to strengthen the information that people have received. . . . So we would like to make a change. . . . Because normally, [the information] would come to us from people who are coming from the lowlands. And they will spend just a few days, and they are under pressure, and they are leaving, and, you know, it's just like throwing a stone into the sea, you know?

The Monatsi's experience reinforces that while churches have been at the forefront of caring for people living with HIV, they have been late to adequately address AIDS in their parishes. It also highlights the potential for both positive and negative contributions to AIDS education and stigma as well as the need for prolonged community engagement.

Chiefs are also influential in shaping local responses to social problems. The kingdom and the chiefdom still have considerable real and symbolic importance for Basotho in resolving problems and establishing social norms. Chiefs hold nonelected paid positions under the Ministry of Local Government and Chieftainship. They are divided into three tiers: principal chiefs (responsible for an entire district), area chiefs (responsible for 10 or more villages), and village chiefs. They fulfill administrative responsibilities at the principal and area levels and provide important social mediation and ceremonial officiating in villages. Caregivers often sought their village chief's permission to send children to the MCS safe home, where they would arrive with a hand-written referral from the chief. Chiefs were also frequently called upon to mediate discussions among kin about caregiver rights. The continued importance of the chieftainship is a reflection of Basotho's embeddedness within kinship networks, clans, and villages. As a fundamental part of Basotho social networks, the structured nature of the chieftainship would be ideal for rolling out AIDS education. Although one of the ministry's goals is "to contribute towards prevention, treatment and

mitigating the impact of HIV and AIDS" (Lesotho Ministry of Local Government and Chieftainship 2012), the widespread impact of this effort was not
evident in Mokhotlong. Some of the caregivers I spoke with said that they had
attended an HIV-centric community meeting (or *pitso*) organized by a chief, but
these efforts were spotty at best and lacked the necessary follow-up, consistency,
and depth.

I spoke at length with Ntate Puseletso, a local village chief, about his role in
the community, including his role as an AIDS educator. I met him through MCS,
where he served on the organization's local board. After observing board meetings, however, I did not get the impression that he or the other board members
were particularly active in educating the community about HIV prevention
or treatment. At one meeting, for example, the board members spent most of
their time discussing whether they should get name tags made for the meetings,
although they all knew each other well, given that they were prominent leaders
in a small community. When I asked Ntate Puseletso about his role in mitigating the impact of HIV/AIDS in his villages, he knew the politicized language of
development efforts but was vague in terms of his actual accomplishments: "Oh,
we do the normal things. Quite a lot, really. Because we work hard for the welfare
of our villages. That is inclusive of health issues, HIV, et cetera. Like, here, for
instance, I have done quite a lot of things regarding HIV/AIDS in order to help
my community. I did trainings on . . . training of, um, teachers of HIV. I'm the
trainer there. I've done a lot on counseling. I've also done a lot on communication for change. Change for communication. In fact, quite a lot of things, really."

Chiefs were often key in organizing their constituents into support groups or
in gathering people into a *pitso* so that others could share information with them.
Since my work was primarily with caregivers of AIDS orphans, I did not observe
or interview chiefs frequently, but I did interact with them regularly. In order to
avoid overstepping cultural bounds, I would usually visit the chief of a village
before talking to residents, particularly when I was collecting household survey
data. I also happened upon *pitsos* a number of times, though never ones pertain-
ing to health. Chiefs' actual involvement in promoting AIDS education and support varied greatly, with some participating regularly in community events and
others never referring a single client to MCS. Chiefs, like pastors, possess both
the necessary authority and cultural knowledge to help improve AIDS education, yet a coordinated and consistent effort to harness that potential has yet to
be realized in Mokhotlong.

In contrast to the informal AIDS education provided by local cultural and
religious institutions, formal AIDS education is now a regular part of school
curricula. Education is positively correlated with HIV/AIDS knowledge (Glick
and Sahn 2007), and as primary education is now free in Lesotho, most young
people attend school until they are at least 12 or 13. At the local high school in

Mokhotlong where my husband, Will, worked, students were required to take a life-skills class, which included AIDS education. Young people are the target of numerous AIDS education and prevention programs across Africa (Obasi et al. 2006; Parsitau 2009; Esu-Williams et al. 2006; Campbell et al. 2005), yet they continue to contract HIV at high rates (Lesotho Ministry of Health 2015). A simple scale-up of interventions to improve AIDS education is insufficient—any response needs to be adjusted to address the localized, social implications of AIDS knowledge and associated behavioral changes.

## CONCEPTIONS AND MISCONCEPTIONS OF HIV/AIDS

The multiple sources that inform Basotho's AIDS knowledge, in conjunction with the tendency to focus on observable symptoms of illness, result in a fractured and fluctuating understanding of the physical implications of HIV infection. Many caregivers and mothers I spoke with were either living with HIV themselves, caring for an HIV-positive child, or had cared for their sons and daughters during the late stages of their illness. Many had attended adherence sessions and frequently visited clinics for checkups and antiretroviral therapy. One would then expect a fairly nuanced understanding of HIV's impact on the body, yet this was not the case. In their explanations of HIV, Basotho tended to fuse their own experiences with what they had learned from multiple competing information sources into a distorted biosocial view of AIDS's impact on the body. My purpose here is not to reinforce stereotyped notions about rural Africans' ignorance regarding health issues; rather, it is to highlight the ineffectiveness of AIDS education in providing people with clear and reliable information. The existing sources of information—which would allow rural Basotho to address the impact of HIV on networks of kin and care in lifesaving ways—are currently inadequate.

When asked to describe someone's illness, Basotho almost never name the illness but instead focus on symptoms the patient is experiencing—especially when discussing HIV, whose common symptoms included pain in the chest and feet, a swollen body and stomach, diarrhea, vomiting, and wasting. This reluctance to name is a reflection not only of a symptom-focused perspective of illness but of a strategy employed by Basotho to avoid stigmatizing loved ones or threatening networks of care. The emphasis on symptoms helps Basotho normalize HIV as something that is "like any other disease"—a phrase I heard repeatedly. Ntate Kanelo claimed that HIV changes the color of the body and can cause mouth sores—referring to oral thrush, a common opportunistic infection associated with HIV, particularly in breastfeeding children. Ntate Kalasi, an HIV-positive father of five, knew that HIV was contracted sexually and so extrapolated that it affected the male and female "parts." 'M'e Maphonolo said that she knew her aunt was HIV positive based on her symptoms: "I have seen the symptoms that she was positive because I have heard that when people have diarrhea, and it doesn't stop, even when people are getting sick and having a headache, and this goes together with diarrhea, they have *that* disease." Like many others, 'M'e Maphonolo's view of HIV relied on symptom observation and was shaped by word-of-mouth accounts. The reliance on physical symptoms confused 77-year-old 'M'e Mamorena as to whether her daughter was actually suffering from HIV. She said, "I didn't see anything when I was washing her. They said I should look at her hair. They said when it's thin like that, she had *that* disease. I said, 'I don't know.' When I looked at her body, I didn't see anything." Her inability to observe symptoms made her doubt the existence of the illness. However, after her daughter passed away, she got herself tested just in case she had contracted the virus while caring for her.

Although the majority of caregivers focused on visible signs of HIV infection, some mentioned its effect on the blood. On numerous occasions, I was told that HIV infection causes "unclean" blood, and a few caregivers mentioned wearing gloves while caring for the sick so that if they had a cut, their blood would not "meet" with someone else's. Ntate Kapo, one of the more knowledgeable caregivers I encountered, said that HIV is "when the veins are not working properly," and it "stops people's blood, and the blood is not clean." When I asked him what happened once you contracted HIV, he surmised, "I think it sucks all the blood, and that person will end up having no blood at all." Given the symbolic importance of blood in reckoning kin relations (recall the expression *mali a llelana*, or "blood cries for blood"), the prospect of losing all of one's blood is both physically and socially traumatic.

Some caregivers were able to articulate, in symptomatic terms, the basic relationship between HIV and AIDS. Those who had attended the adherence sessions generally understood that AIDS was more severe than HIV, but they were not able to explicitly connect AIDS with a lowered CD4 count or the inability for the immune system to fight illness in the body. 'M'e Maliehi expressed this vague understanding well: "The most dangerous is AIDS. And HIV is when someone is infected. I don't know how to show the difference." Ntate Kalasi said that he understood the difference between HIV and AIDS like this: "I heard that when you have HIV, you have a small illness. But when you have AIDS, you have to take the big pills. . . . You are still powerful when you have HIV." Ntate Kalasi is himself HIV positive, but as of September 2009, he had not yet initiated ART. His understanding of HIV reflected his own view of his illness as "small" and himself as "powerful." Kotsi's grandfather, Ntate Kapo, described the qualitative difference between HIV and AIDS but also told me that the drugs could cure HIV: "The difference of HIV is infection only. And AIDS is something else. I have heard that people who have AIDS don't survive. People who have HIV can be cured if they take the drugs." The confusion among people like Ntate Kapo, who attended three adherence sessions when his grandson was starting treatment, indicates a need for the clarification and reinforcement of key issues to deepen patients' and caregivers' comprehension.

Even while HIV was normalized as an illness "like any other," most people understood that there was no cure—the point was hammered home in adherence sessions. Yet many were still optimistic about the future. 'M'e Mamorena used the analogy of tying a rope to describe how the medication helped her granddaughter Hopolang: "They have tied it. I see that this thing was going to be increased if she was not given drugs. She was given drugs while she was still young. Now it's stable." I asked 'M'e Maliapeng, the HIV-positive caregiver for two young girls, what she learned at her adherence sessions. She replied, "Ah, I asked them whether after taking the pills the infection will go away. They said no. But the virus will not have power to work on my body." Others had experienced such visible and tangible success with ART that people had hope that a full biomedical cure was forthcoming. 'M'e Mapoloko witnessed a dramatic change in her grandson, Joki, and told me that there was a cure "if you are using the pills in a good way." Ntate Kapo also witnessed his grandson, Kotsi, recover from near death after initiating ART. Like 'M'e Mamorena, he said that the drugs "have stopped it," and he thought that Kotsi was cured. Multiple conflicting sources of information were likely responsible for this confusion. When Lebo's grandmother was informed (incorrectly) that his HIV status was no longer positive, she interpreted this not as an error in the original diagnosis (or in the rediagnosis, as was the case) but as that his HIV had come and gone. Her bewilderment throughout this saga of multiple and conflicting diagnoses reinforced her tenuous understanding of how HIV impacts the body and how treatment works to fight the virus.

Many caregivers also held fundamental misconceptions about the nature of HIV. There are still some, especially among the elderly, who question HIV's true identity, attributing it instead to locally defined illnesses such as *kokoana* and *mokaola*, which have been around for decades and have similar clusters of symptoms. Yet this does not necessarily prevent people from adhering to recommended treatments. As opposed to having Sesotho origins, one young HIV-positive widow and mother said that she heard people in her community say that "AIDS is the disease made by *makhooa*," though she claims that she did not personally believe this and thought all Basotho should be tested. 'M'e Malefu, a village health worker, said, "Some are talking about the things that are not true. Like me, the first time when I heard about it, I thought maybe some black people have met some people with whom their blood did not go together. And

I thought that this disease came from there." 'M'e Malefu expressed uncertainty about where HIV comes from despite her training and exposure to people living with HIV, with whom she worked closely.

In other cases, misinformation led to confusing ideas about transmission and prevention that could have serious consequences for dependent children and the success of planned intervention strategies. For example, 24-year-old 'M'e Matsiu told me a complicated story about HIV being caused by women having too many abortions. She then added, "And they sleep with someone who has not been washed, and later they will say, 'That person has *mahae* [a locally defined type of vaginal discharge].' And when they go to the doctor, those *mahae* go out from their female organs. And when they get tested, they are found positive." A common rumor was also that HIV was caused by the buffer used in HIV testing and that condoms had worms that caused HIV. In all of these examples, informal information networks led to varying and often contradictory misconceptions about HIV that impacted decision-making by patients and caregivers and increased the risk of infection and treatment failure.

When visiting caregivers, if they demonstrated a gap in knowledge that would impact their health or the health of their child, I would ask if they had questions or wanted clarifications. I found myself on many occasions explaining the progression from HIV to AIDS and the connection between CD4 count and the body's inability to fight off infection. Caregivers frequently indicated a willingness to learn and a desire for biomedical information about the disease, demonstrating that other service providers were not adequately addressing their needs or offering a venue where they could comfortably ask essential questions.

## ELDERLY CAREGIVERS AND HIV/AIDS

Elderly people in Lesotho are often poorly informed about HIV/AIDS compared to younger members of the community. In part, this is because they are not targeted for prevention and testing, as they are predominantly beyond their sexual prime and are therefore less likely to contract the illness.[2] However, given that the elderly—particularly grandmothers—are primarily responsible for the care of orphans, community-based responses are needed to reduce the knowledge gap between the young and elderly.

The elderly view HIV/AIDS, somewhat correctly, as a young person's disease. For most young Basotho, HIV is a lived reality that has always been a part of their public health consciousness. In contrast, elderly Basotho bring with them a history of interactions with illness and public health initiatives that color and shape their understandings of this newest health crisis. Matseli's grandfather, Ntate Kanelo, said that many people were infected because of sex. His wife, 'M'e Maliehi, responded, "I don't know what causes that for young people. It is true that even old people have it—but not like young people." 'M'e Masekha, Thapo's grandmother, also equated sexual risk with younger people. She told me that young people should use condoms when having sex. When my research assistant, Ausi Ntsoaki, asked whether she should also use condoms, she replied sheepishly, "No, 'M'e. I'm no longer doing that, since 2001." Those who were sexually active were more reluctant to use condoms because, as 'M'e Mapoloko said, "we have not grown up using those things." Yet the current population of HIV-positive adults is living longer because of ART, adding a new dimension to the management of the disease. New health problems are emerging as the challenges of HIV are amplified by chronic illnesses associated with old age (Negin, Mills, and Albone 2011; Negin and Cumming 2010). The near absence of HIV programs targeting elderly people in southern Africa ignores the real risks and challenges they face as both patients and caregivers.

The elderly residents of Mokhotlong often expressed denial and discomfort when talking about HIV. While misinformation and knowledge gaps posed real problems, many who appeared to know very little were often masking discomfort with the subject, insecurity about the validity of their knowledge, and a desire to disconnect the illness from their networks of kin and care. When I first asked about HIV, many elderly caregivers would agree to discuss it but distanced themselves from the disease by claiming that they knew very little. 'M'e Mapoloko, the primary caregiver for HIV-positive Joki, told me, "There is nothing I know." Nkhabu's great-grandmother, 'M'e Marefiloe, also denied knowing anything. I told her just to answer as best she could, and she replied, "I don't want to lie." However, over the course of our discussions, they both revealed a deeper knowledge than they had first let on.

In the following conversation, 'M'e Matlotliso, Kotsi's blind and elderly great-grandmother, exposed her discomfort with discussing HIV and her insecurity about the veracity of her HIV knowledge while also revealing the pervasiveness of informal conversations about HIV in the community.

ELLEN: Have you heard people talk about HIV and AIDS?

'M'E MATLOTLISO: *Ache*, no, 'M'e, because I haven't gone to the clinic. I have heard people saying, "AIDS, AIDS, AIDS," and I'm always asking them, "What is it, this disease? Where does it appear from on the person?" *Kannete*. I don't know it [*laughs*]. . . . I know that it's a disease, but I don't know it. And I'm always asking them, every day, to tell me what it is. [*Laughs*]

ELLEN: From what you know, do you think it's a big problem in Lesotho?

'M'E MATLOTLISO: Yes, they say it makes Basotho suffer, when I hear them.

ELLEN: Do you know how people get HIV?

'M'E MATLOTLISO: Ah ah, I don't know. That's why I'm saying I'm always asking them to tell me.

ELLEN: Oh. Do you know anyone who has HIV?

'M'E MATLOTLISO: Ah ah. I don't know at all. [The neighbors] just talk about it. Saying this and this and this, but I don't hear what they are talking about. Mmm. I've just heard people, but they are not talking to me, saying some have run away from the clinic, what and what and what, maybe they have AIDS, and they run away when they are told to do something at the clinic. So ah . . .

ELLEN: *Nkhono*, do you want to know what HIV is?

'M'E MATLOTLISO: *Ache*, 'M'e, no.

It is unclear whether 'M'e Matlotliso actually knew very little about HIV. Although her great-grandson was HIV positive, he lived with his grandfather ('M'e Matlotliso's son) in an adjacent home. With her limited mobility and vision, she may not have witnessed him taking his medication twice daily. However, she likely knew that he visited the clinic with his grandfather every month or perhaps overheard his grandfather calling for him at seven in the morning and evening each day to take his medications. It seems unlikely that she knew as little as she claimed, but she clearly had no interest in discussing the matter with me, in contrast to the many other topics on which she liked to hold forth.

Like 'M'e Matlotliso, other caregivers claimed ignorance at first but over time revealed extensive knowledge and deeply held beliefs about HIV transmission, treatment, and prevention. When I told 'M'e Mamorena, the great-grandmother and primary caregiver for HIV-positive Hopolang, that I wanted to ask her what she knew about HIV, she responded, "I won't answer. I don't know it. It's my first time to hear about it this year." 'M'e Mamorena did not attend adherence sessions for Hopolang because she was unable to reach the clinic due to severe arthritis in her knees and back. However, it would be nearly impossible for even the most remote villager not to know about HIV until 2008, as the rate of infection at that time had held steady at around 23 percent for a decade. 'M'e Mamorena had been caring for Hopolang for several years and for her own infected daughter (Hopolang's grandmother) prior to her death in 2008. Uncharacteristically, on one visit, she did not shy away from addressing the issue head on. She told me that she frequently heard young people talking about the disease: "I'm always asking, 'What is this AIDS?'" Yet because it is associated with sex, she said that people told her, "Ah, *nkhono*, it's not a disease that you can know." Nonetheless, she chose to get an HIV test in 2008 after her daughter passed away: "They said she had AIDS. Her hair was thin. She was thin. When I was washing her, they were giving me some gloves. At the end, I saw that I was not able to work with them. I was touching her with my bare hands, and they said I will have AIDS, and I went to get tested again. There was nothing. I said, 'I don't know this thing.'" Her loving care of her daughter is even more powerful given that she clearly held some awareness about the disease and its transmission through fluids. Yet her explanation for her decision to test also indicates confusion about the risk of infection and ongoing gossip and stigma in the community.

Unlike her original assertion that she knew nothing about HIV/AIDS, 'M'e Mamorena ultimately revealed a great deal of both information and misinformation. She knew that HIV was transmitted sexually and that treatment is for life, but it is not a cure. She said that everyone should go for counseling and know their status. She had also heard that condoms prevented HIV but wanted to know if they harbored worms that caused the virus. She mentioned two Sesotho illnesses and was unsure if they were synonymous with AIDS. The first, *mofetse*, she described as a disease suffered by women that causes soft bones. The second, *mokaola*, she described as causing sores on the chest and a black rash. At first, she told me that people were wrong to say that *mokaola* was the same as AIDS, but she later admitted that she was unsure. In contrast, her great-granddaughter, five-year-old Hopolang, with the help of her 10-year-old sister, was able to follow her complicated and ever-changing ART regimen. 'M'e Mamorena proudly boasted about her granddaughter's knowledge:

> When it's time for her to take the pills, she will be calling Ntate Khosoane [to see his clock]. If Ntate Khosoane can say it's seven, she will come back to the house running, saying, "Bring my pills, my pills." And she knows that she's supposed to take the full pill in the morning, and in the evening, she's supposed to take the half. And she will be saying, "Give me half, half, half, half." She knows them exactly. Even her medicines, she will be asking for the teaspoon [of Bactrim].[3] The problem is in the morning, when she is in a hurry to go to school, she just runs to school.

Even after telling me all this, when I later asked her what she thought *mokaola* was, she replied, "I think it's that HIV that I don't know." 'M'e Mamorena's denial was, at least in part, a coping mechanism that she employed to protect the close and loving relationship she had with her great-granddaughter, whom she also relied on for help.

Many elderly caregivers linked AIDS and *mokaola*, the sexually transmitted Sesotho illness, as a way of connecting current experiences and knowledge with their past. This incorporation of the strange into the familiar is what social psychologist Serge Moscovici calls "anchoring," which provides a way of making sense of foreign and potentially dangerous things by "reduc[ing] them to ordinary categories and images, to set them in a familiar context" (Moscovici 2001, 42). *Mokaola* was described to me as having a wide variety of symptoms, including genital sores, genital discharge, thinned hair, and body rashes (described alternatively as all over the body, small, and black). Ntate Kapo said that a person who had *mokaola* was "bitten." When HIV first appeared in the community, many adults had heard that it was not new at all but rather *mokaola*, which had been around for years. Although attributing a rise in HIV to a well-known local illness gave it continuity and helped people make sense of it, it also created confusion and perpetuated AIDS denialism. Ntate Kapo said when HIV first appeared, he heard other people refute its existence: "There is no such thing here. They were saying that. Saying, '*Mmm-mmm*. This is not HIV.' They were saying it's *mokaola*. They say it's the disease that we know—same as in the past." 'M'e Marefiloe told me that many people now understand that what Basotho are suffering from is in fact HIV, not *mokaola*. I asked her what she thought, and she said, "I don't know. . . . Now that it has an English name, I don't know anything about it." It was easier to connect to the illness when it resonated with her past experiences.

The isolation of elderly caregivers in Mokhotlong from accurate biomedical knowledge and support networks is of grave concern. Grandmothers continue to bear the brunt of caregiving responsibilities that stem from AIDS mortality and orphaning. They perform essential, lifesaving tasks such as administering complicated drug regimens and taking dependent adults and children to the clinic or hospital when needed. Elderly people in Lesotho are also respected as important leaders in their communities, both informally and in official capacities such as religious leaders and chiefs. Thus elderly Basotho could act as an established and trustworthy source of guidance for the rest of the community. Educating elderly Basotho could be an important step in improving care for AIDS patients and strengthening AIDS education for younger generations of Basotho.

## WHERE PREVENTION MEETS KINSHIP

Basotho regularly encounter educational and biomedical interventions designed to prevent the spread of HIV between sexual partners and between mother and child, but local responses to prevention efforts have been mixed, as evidenced by the slow decline in the number of new infections in the region (Kelly et al. 2006; UNAIDS 2017). Implementation of the popular ABC model (Abstinence, Be Faithful, Condomize)—which targets behavior change—is widespread, yet scholarly responses to this approach are mixed. Proponents of the ABC model, including anthropologist Ted Green, argue that this approach, which has worked in Uganda, is simple and empowers individuals to protect their own health as they wait for governments and NGOs to address other social and structural drivers of the pandemic (Green 2003; Green et al. 2006). Critics argue that the ABC method has been less effective because it fails to address the biocultural aspects of HIV (Parker 2001; Farmer 2003).

Prevention efforts intersect most directly with kinship networks in three ways: condom use, partner fidelity, and the prevention of mother-to-child transmission (PMTCT). All three of these prevention areas threaten basic social relationships because they implicate not only the nature and strength of these relationships but the fundamental definitions of what it means to be a wife, a husband, a mother, and a caregiver. Each of these prevention areas also sheds light on culturally constructed notions of gender and sexuality and the ways in which married women in particular have limited ability to protect themselves from contracting HIV. In the following, I explore each of these areas of prevention, as they shed light on the explicit and implicit tensions that exist between sociality and health.

## Condoms

Condom use has been the primary focus of prevention efforts across Africa for the simple reason that condoms are inexpensive, easy to distribute, and easy to use. However, interventions that ignore the cultural implications of condom use for both men and women have largely failed (Campbell et al. 2005; Booth 2004). My own data confirm that, on their own, condoms are not a reliable HIV-prevention method for Mokhotlong residents. Condom use threatens the strength of marriage by drawing attention to infidelity and by denying the possibility of conception in a culture where parenthood remains an important rite of passage and symbol of status and happiness. Rumors, jokes, and an often-expressed male dislike for condoms mask the underlying social implications of condom use on marriage, parenthood, and gendered power imbalances.

The Sesotho word for condom is *khohlopo*, which means "gumboot."[4] Basotho also refer to condoms using the English word but more often adopt the slang "CD" (perhaps as a way of avoiding embarrassment). For those living close to town, inconsistent condom use is not an issue of availability, since male condoms are widely distributed. Condoms are free at clinics, hospitals, government offices, and even on a small table next to the ATM in Mokhotlong or in a box nailed to the side of a rural village health worker's rondavel. They can also be purchased at local shops and grocery stores. Female condoms are not nearly as ubiquitous but are occasionally available at clinics and hospitals. At a village health-worker training session that I attended, every attendee received a box of several hundred condoms to hand out in their communities. I once saw the driver of a government truck toss boxes of condoms out his window to locals who were temporarily employed to fix a section of flooded road.

One challenge of measuring condom usage, however, is that the only indication of use is through personal reporting. As 'M'e Nthabiseng said, "I think health issues are always complicated and not easy to measure. Because, for instance, if you want people to protect themselves, and you give them condoms, you are never going to see if they use them. All they will do, they will tell you [that they are using them]." People may report condom use, and even though they may use condoms sometimes, they may not use them every time. Lesotho's 2014 demographic health survey (Lesotho Ministry of Health 2016) found that only 65 percent of men and 54 percent of women who had two or more sexual partners in the past year had used a condom during their most recent sexual intercourse. As expected, condom usage for married women was very low (17 percent), and education and urban residence were both positively correlated with condom use (Lesotho Ministry of Health 2016). A more accurate measure of the likelihood of consistent condom usage is reflected in Basotho's attitudes about condoms, which range from positive acceptance regarding their preventive usefulness to suspicion and outright dislike. Their mixed feelings about condoms and condom use point to their inconsistency and unreliability as an HIV-prevention method.

The majority of Mokhotlong residents I spoke to, both young and old, knew that condoms were intended to prevent HIV infection, though some questioned their efficacy. When I asked 'M'e Maliapeng what she would tell her young niece when she was older about HIV prevention, she told me, "Hmm! This one is difficult. Because the girls like to disobey; even if you have told them what not to do, they don't listen to you. It's better if we encourage them to use condoms." Premarital sex, while discouraged in theory, bears no real social sanction in Mokhotlong. When 'M'e Maliapeng said that she would not expect her niece to listen when she told her "what not do to" (i.e., have sex), she did at least think that she might be convinced to use a condom.

In contrast, religious leaders like Ntate Monatsi preached the importance of abstinence. When I asked him about condom use, he told me that he only encouraged it among married couples: "Ah, condom, yeah, it is recommended. We are ready to teach about condom in the church to encourage people who are in marriage but have tested and could be running the risk of infection. So there we believe that the use of condom is fine. But people who are not in marriage. Ah, abstinence. Yes. Yeah." Ntate Monatsi, though, was skeptical of consistent condom use: "Well, one realizes—looking at the infection rate and death rate and how, you know, people are sick—you really can wonder if a condom is even making any difference. I don't think people are using the condom." Although he was willing to state that condoms were not widely used, he avoided the implication of infidelity that condom use inside marriage implied.

Positive attitudes toward condoms, however, did not appear to translate into consistent and widespread condom usage in practice, particularly among young and married people. I visited 'M'e Maphonolo, the young HIV-positive mother of three and caregiver of her two orphaned brothers, in the middle of the day, one June, while her youngest daughter was napping. She was washing clothes in a dark-green basin in her dimly lit rondavel, absentmindedly pushing denim around gray soapy water. She told me that she encouraged her friends to use condoms but confirmed that usage was inconsistent. She described a scenario where a close friend was seeking her advice because her boyfriend did not want to use condoms during sex: "I said, 'You should leave him.' I always encourage that if they refuse to use condoms, they should leave them because they don't know whether [their partner] has it [HIV] or not. They also don't know if they have it or not. No one is telling each other. It's better if you leave them." She also suggested that the spread of misinformation made condom negotiation difficult. She told me, "Some of them, they don't like the way they are. They hate that oily stuff [lubricant]. They are saying, 'Where is it coming from, and what is it for?' They just think they are the ones causing the disease. And if you don't believe [in HIV], you will listen to them." Here 'M'e Maphonolo touches on one of the circular paradoxes of HIV prevention. HIV is stigmatized, so people are unwilling to disclose their status, which makes it difficult to negotiate condom use, which leads to new HIV infections, which results in more HIV stigmatization. Although she was not explicitly advocating abstinence, 'M'e Maphonolo believed that her friend should not stay with a man who was unwilling to use a condom or disclose his HIV status—yet many people do neither of those. This presents limited choices for young, sexually active Basotho both inside of marriage and out.

In addition to the social difficulties of negotiating condom use even among those who believe in their efficacy, many rumors about condoms cause confusion and distrust. One of the most common myths I heard was that condoms cause HIV infections. As already described, many people repeated the rumor that condoms contained worms and that these worms could pass from one person to another during intercourse. Kwansa (2014) found that in Ghana, the worm metaphor was commonly used by health professionals to avoid discussing HIV by its real name, leaving space for nonbiomedical causality. I was often told that if I boiled a condom and put it out in the sun, I could see it for myself, though when pressed, nobody had witnessed this firsthand. Ausi Ntsoaki and I decided to perform this experiment. We boiled a condom for 30 minutes and left it in the sun for over an hour. Of course, nothing unusual happened, and we were able report in future conversations that this was false, as we had witnessed it for ourselves. When I told this to 'M'e Masenate, she replied, "Yes, I'm always asking myself whether it is the truth or not. And I wasn't sure, and I didn't know who will tell me the truth." Although she doubted the veracity of the rumor, she expressed difficulty in finding reliable information.

'M'e Karabo, a young VCT officer from the hospital, occasionally had lunch with me on the lawn of the Mokhotlong Hospital. While we munched *makoenya* (fat cakes), she told me about the wide range of condom-related complaints she heard during her counseling sessions, especially from men. Some men said that they experienced pain in their kidneys or liver while using condoms, which she dismissed as untrue. Some said that condoms did not fit their penises, while others complained that "they can't feel" while using condoms. As an explanation for why men did not like condoms, people often repeated the well-known expression "You can't eat wrapped sweets," relying on disarming humor as a method of dismissal.

Men's distaste for condoms is closely linked to women's lack of power in negotiating condom use, particularly with their husbands. Married women are among the most at risk for HIV infection, in part because condom negotiation between married partners is even more difficult than between unmarried partners (Clark 2004). Many of the Basotho women I spoke with agreed that it would be difficult to ask one's husband to use a condom. The newly married 'M'e Masenate addressed the question hypothetically: "I don't think it's possible if you have your husband, unless you are still sleeping with other men—you can use them. But not with your husband. . . . Because sometimes the parents-in-law will say they want children. And you will not have children if you are using CDs." Marriage and childbearing decisions are not merely left to the whims of the couple but are subject to the expectations and desires of the extended family. If a woman asks her husband to use a condom, she is not only denying the possibility of a child but also implicitly expressing her suspicions of his infidelity or alluding to her own. In this context, men's stated preference for condom-free sex and women's acceptance of it allows them both to avoid difficult conversations that could lead to marital dissolution.

One young teacher—a friend and colleague of Will's from the high school—was separated from her husband. He had left for Durban (in South Africa) three years prior, while she was pregnant with their second child, and never returned. She had been saving money to find him and bring him home, but she worried that she would not be able to protect herself if successful. She tearfully told Will and me over lunch one day that she was worried that she would contract HIV because she feared that he had been sleeping with prostitutes. She was grappling with the conundrum of trying to reunite her family—which would have powerful emotional, material, and social benefits—while at the same time protecting her health. 'M'e Karabo, the VCT counselor at the hospital, confirmed that many women have trouble negotiating condom use with their husbands. She told me that women "are always coming here to ask for our assistance to talk to their husbands," and she counseled them on the goodness (bohlokoa) of condom use, even within marriage. If a seropositive couple wanted to conceive a child, 'M'e Karabo encouraged them to work with the doctor to ensure that their CD4 counts were high and to determine the best time to conceive, using condoms during the balance of the month. 'M'e Karabo told me that because her husband worked in South Africa, they used condoms but would employ this strategy when they decided to have a baby. The strategic use of condoms is particularly important for serodiscordant couples,[5] but it also helps prevent reinfection between seropositive partners, which can accelerate the onset of AIDS (Schiltz and Sandfort 2000; Gottlieb et al. 2004).

Condom use has the potential to be one of the most effective methods of preventing HIV transmission because of their cost, ease of use, and effectiveness. Basotho generally acknowledge that condoms prevent HIV, and many state that, at least in theory, they are useful as a protective method. However, inconsistent condom use and pervasive misinformation pose significant obstacles, even among young men and women, who are generally well versed in HIV prevention. Married couples rely on familiar tropes about the dangers and displeasures of condoms as a tactic to avoid facing the social implications of using them. Women in particular are left with a difficult choice: they can attempt to protect themselves, potentially causing marital strife and denying the possibility of a child, or they can risk their long-term health to maintain social networks.

## Partner Infidelity

In addition to the importance of condom use, partner fidelity has been a major focus of prevention efforts in the region. Like condoms, "faithfulness" is not a straightforward prevention method; it gets at the heart of people's intimate relationships, cultural attitudes about concurrent partnerships, and structural barriers to fidelity such as long-term migrant labor. Public health messages stress the importance of "one love," or faithfulness to one's spouse or primary partner, in an attempt to combat the cultural expectation demonstrated in the Sesotho idiom "Monna ke mokopu oa nama" (Men are like pumpkins, spreading everywhere). Men and women both uphold fidelity in marriage as the ideal while also expressing the expectation that their partners—especially men—will have difficulty adhering to this standard.

During one long drive out to visit an MCS client, two young female outreach workers insisted that more than 80 percent of men cheated on their wives. One of the women was married with two young children, while the other, who was HIV positive, claimed that this was the reason she never wanted to get married at all. Instead, she had a son with her long-term boyfriend, whose marriage proposals she regularly rebuffed. Of course, this statistic is pure speculation on their part, but it indicates their concerns as young women in Lesotho and reinforces the cultural belief in men's infidelity. 'M'e Matlai, the young teacher whose husband went to South Africa and did not return, told me, "Here people have many partners. It is so bad. This life encourages the disease." Most women I spoke with focused on male infidelity, but 'M'e Matlai acknowledged that both men and women have sexual relationships outside of marriage. However, she viewed men as the catalyst for this behavior because they "leave their wives inside the house" and go look for other women. She told me that women were unfaithful because they needed something that their husbands were not providing, or they were lonely because they had been abandoned by their husbands. If men changed their behavior, she told me, women would also change.

A few individuals recognized the broader structural factors that contributed to infidelity; however, they were community leaders and educators who had received special training in HIV prevention and education. Ntate and 'M'e Monatsi, the pastors who had increased efforts in their church to educate their parishioners about HIV, said that people were making "a small change" when it came to fidelity, but family separation due to migrant labor made this difficult. In addition to being a pastor, Ntate Monatsi sold coffins and transported home the bodies of Basotho who passed away in South Africa while at work. Again, pointing to men's inability to resist temptation, he explained, "You know there is stubbornness, especially from the men's side, because there are so many women working on the farms. Yeah, they outnumber men." 'M'e Matlai, a peer educator, said that the situation could be improved if there were more employment opportunities in Lesotho. She astutely noted that "a major problem of HIV is this problem of poverty." Speaking from personal experience, 'M'e Karabo, the VCT counselor, expressed that it was difficult to remain faithful when a couple was separated because of work. She worried that her husband, who frequently took month-long trips to South Africa for work, was not able to remain faithful to her. She lamented, "What makes my relationship difficult is this arrangement. Because I know a man is not like a woman. When he feels that [desire], he just meets [has sex with] a person. Mine I control. I can tell myself, no, I'm waiting for my husband, while he's not waiting for me."

Many people suggested that faithfulness was a key factor in HIV prevention, though few provided any insight as to how this might be achieved. Ntate Kanelo offered, "I should stay at my house, and not go to other people's." People often used such expressions as "visit" or "meet" as euphemisms for sex. Tsepiso's mother, who is HIV positive, simply told me that "people should stop having sex," although she no doubt recognized this as untenable. 'M'e Nthabiseng worried that the effectiveness of HIV treatment would only exacerbate infidelity: "Ah, I think people will continue to have new infections. I don't see people really changing to the situation, where they are like, 'Oh no, we have to stop new infections.' Now that they have ARVs, they see people coping. It's like they found an answer. HIV, it's going to take a while to really—for new infections to be lower. The way people do things, behavior-wise, aahhh, I don't know."

So far, 'M'e Nthabiseng is correct. Basotho are living longer because of ART, but new infections are declining slowly because of low comprehensive knowledge about HIV, early onset of sexual activity, low condom use, and multiple sexual partners. In 2014, there were 17,000 new HIV infections in Lesotho, down only 29 percent from 2001, missing the targeted 50 percent HIV-incidence reduction by a wide margin (Lesotho Ministry of Health 2015). The expected reduction of new infections that public health experts hoped would come with the widespread availability of ART has been stalled because only 57 percent of all people living with HIV know their status, and only 46 percent of all people living with HIV have access to ARVs (UNAIDS 2016).

It is difficult to assess, both from my own fieldwork and existing literature, the frequency of extramarital sexual encounters in the region. In Lesotho, 7 percent of all women and 27 percent of all men reported having two or more concurrent partnerships, likely a low estimate due to underreporting (Lesotho Ministry of Health 2016). Some scholars warn that a focus on male infidelity misses the frequency of female infidelity, often within transactional partnerships where gifts or cash provide women with some agency in accessing resources (Hunter 2002; Kaufman 2004; Leclerc-Madlala 2003). Others argue that it is not necessarily the number of sexual partners but the overlapping nature of multiple concurrent partnerships that has facilitated the spread of HIV (Epstein 2007; Mah and Halperin 2010). Women with multiple concurrent partnerships are frequently unmarried, but young married women remain the highest at-risk group for HIV infection. Parikh (2007) argues that public health messages condemning extramarital affairs in Uganda have had the unintended consequence of creating secrecy among married partners regarding their extramarital relationships, thus putting married women at greater risk of infection because they cannot protect themselves by knowing when their husbands are unfaithful. In Lesotho, men and women agree that faithfulness in relationships is important but unrealistic, and the expectation of infidelity in combination with inconsistent condom use limits the ability for both men and women to protect themselves from acquiring HIV from their long-term partners.

One of the paradoxes of increased attention to partner fidelity is that an already frowned-upon, albeit accepted, practice—infidelity—is now further fraught with the blame and stigma of HIV infection, resulting in increased reluctance to disclose one's HIV status. The joint stigmas of HIV and infidelity thus amplify one another. Admitting infidelity no longer simply means disappointing one's spouse—it can place the blame on the unfaithful partner for infecting his or her spouse and children with a disease that ultimately will kill them. This does not imply that messages regarding faithfulness need to be removed from dialogues about HIV prevention. Rather, prevention efforts must take into account how messages about fidelity may reduce partner communication, decrease the likelihood of disclosure, and increase HIV stigma by making infidelity coterminous with the spread of illness to one's kin.

## Prevention of Mother-to-Child Transmission
The vertical transmission of HIV (from mother to child) is also fraught with stigma, blame, and silence due to the painful ways it implicates mothers in the

illness of their children and threatens the mother-child bond. Although men are also implicated in the HIV status of their children, perhaps even more so, given the higher rates of male infidelity, they are distanced by the pathology of mother-to-child transmission, which can occur in utero, during birth, and through breastfeeding—three important acts of maternal nurturing and shared substance.

Although the majority of my interlocutors were caregivers of orphaned children, I also frequently visited several mothers trying to prevent the vertical transmission of HIV to their unborn or nursing babies. In addition, I observed the delivery of services to PMTCT patients through MCS and during clinic observations. The prevention of mother-to-child transmission is one of the more successful HIV interventions because it is a relatively simple, effective, and inexpensive intervention that capitalizes on well-established antenatal health behaviors. According to the WHO (World Health Organization), without intervention, the risk of mother-to-child transmission ranges from 15 to 45 percent, depending on the viral load of the mother. However, with relatively simple and cost-effective interventions in breastfeeding populations with virtually no access to caesarian sections, the risk of transmission can be reduced to less than 5 percent (WHO 2012).

In 2003, the Lesotho government launched a program aimed specifically at improving PMTCT services, with the ultimate goal of reaching 100 percent of HIV-positive pregnant women during their antenatal clinic visits. According to the Joint United Nations Programme on HIV/AIDS (UNAIDS 2010), PMTCT interventions in Lesotho have resulted in a marked improvement in transmission rates. Between 2004 and 2008, the number of facilities providing PMTCT services in Lesotho went from 9 to 180. In 2004, only 2,764 HIV-positive pregnant women were tested for HIV; 37,159 were tested in 2009. The proportion of pregnant women and newborn infants receiving antiretroviral drugs around the time of birth also increased (UNAIDS 2010). Effective PMTCT has the potential to benefit the current crisis in caregiving by reducing the number of orphans through improved maternal health and lessening the challenges of orphan care associated with HIV-positive children.

The ideal scenario for successful PMTCT in Lesotho is that a woman voluntarily tests for HIV at her first antenatal visit, unless she already knows that she is positive. She begins taking ART immediately;[6] delivers her baby at the hospital, where the infant will receive a short course of ARVs; breastfeeds exclusively for six months; and then introduces food and continues to breastfeed until the child's first birthday. These measures drastically reduce the viral load of the mother during pregnancy and at the time of birth, thereby reducing the chance that she will transmit HIV to her child during labor and ensuring that the child is nourished through the first year. During this time, a woman should carefully monitor her own health and eat a healthy and varied diet. However, numerous structural challenges complicate the realization of this hypothetical scenario. Women often have poor knowledge about their date of conception, and this delays the onset of treatment. They may live far from the hospital, without access to transportation with the onset of labor. Furthermore, HIV-positive women often go into labor early (Steer 2005). Some women anticipate this by going to the hospital around the eighth month of pregnancy to live in the modest huts located at the edge of the hospital grounds reserved for women waiting to deliver. However, this potentially month-long (or more) absence can be problematic for women who have caregiving and other responsibilities at home. Until 2010, when Lesotho began providing the full course of antiretroviral treatment for pregnant women regardless of CD4 count (UNAIDS 2012), the clinics responded to this by giving some women a minimum package, called the Mother/Baby Pack. Introduced in Lesotho in 2007, this package included all the necessary medications and detailed instructions for women to self-administer ARVs until they were able to get to the hospital. However, even while this program was operating, distribution was limited because of supply issues.

In Lesotho, pregnant women regularly visit clinics for antenatal care and did so well before the spread of HIV. This facilitated the implementation of PMTCT services, including HIV testing. In theory, all HIV testing is voluntary (Government of Lesotho 2004); in practice, pregnant women are rarely given a choice, and a woman wishing to avoid testing would have to forego antenatal care altogether. 'M'e Matsiu was tested during her pregnancy as a matter of routine. I asked her if she could have refused if she wanted to, and she said, "I was so afraid.... Because it was my first time to get tested. And I was asking myself what is going to happen. ... I asked them first whether I can refuse or not, and they said no, especially when people are in that condition [pregnant]." 'M'e Mamohato tested during her pregnancy as well. She was also reluctant: "I didn't want to, but they said I must be tested." 'M'e Karabo, the VCT counselor, confirmed the experiences of these women by admitting that she does not give pregnant women a choice: "Now it is a matter of must, for pregnancy." The power structure of patient-caregiver interactions and the pervasive lack of questioning by Basotho patients reinforce this unequal dynamic. This effectively means there is *de facto* mandatory testing for the majority of women of childbearing age.

Women often find out about their HIV status first while receiving antenatal care; it is up to them to convince their male partners to test as well. All of this threatens women's health autonomy and reinforces a gender dynamic where women are made responsible for the health of the family, while men are distanced from their role in the transmission of HIV from mother-to-child. On one occasion, the clinic lost the HIV test results of a young mother who was pregnant with twins. Even though she gave birth at the hospital, she did not receive

PMTCT, and both twins contracted HIV, one dying before her first birthday. Her husband blamed her for their children's sickness, and she faced numerous caregiving challenges due to her daughters' multiple hospitalizations and her husband's lack of support. Ultimately, the couple divorced.

Breastfeeding is one of the most contested areas of mother-to-child transmission due to its position as a highly visible activity central to Basotho's ideas about care and childrearing. Milk is not merely nourishing—it is a key substance that creates important lasting bonds between a mother and child and between siblings (see chapter 1). Exclusive formula feeding is associated with lower HIV rates, but there are numerous barriers to formula feeding: clean water sources are often unreliable (Oladokun, Brown, and Osinusi 2010; Coutsoudis 2001), formula is cost-prohibitive, and the visibility of formula-feeding exposes mothers and children to HIV-related stigma (Doherty 2010). Mixed feeding (a combination of breast milk and formula or other foods and liquids) is not recommended, because it increases the risk of diarrheal disease, malnutrition, and HIV transmission (Coutsoudis 2001). Exclusively breastfed babies are less likely to be exposed to infection, reducing the opportunities for the virus to pass between mother and child. But it is common for Basotho to feed their children sugar water or *lesheshele* (porridge) after they are a few months old, increasing the likelihood that contaminated water or food will weaken their defenses and lead to infection. Accordingly, PMTCT patients are counseled not to practice mixed feeding, although this is difficult to monitor. It is also difficult for mothers—and sometimes health care providers—to keep up with PMTCT recommendations. In 2009, the WHO changed its breastfeeding recommendations from exclusive breastfeeding for six months, followed by rapid weaning, to continued breastfeeding for one year even after other foods are introduced (WHO 2009). The risk of malnutrition drastically increases if a child is weaned rapidly at six months because of the continued importance of milk in the face of food insecurity and the time it takes most babies to transition fully to solid foods. By 2013, some women in Mokhotlong were still abiding by the six-month weaning rule, which had been emphasized to them for years as a way to ensure their babies' survival and was now being linked to increased mortality.

Monitoring exclusive breastfeeding is also a challenge because of the unreliability of self-reporting. Although MCS is one of the few organizations that provide formula under some circumstances (such as if a mother has died or if a woman has multiple births or breastmilk supply issues), 'M'e Nthabiseng worried that for some women, formula would increase the risk of mixed feeding. MCS only provides formula for HIV-positive mothers if they agree to stop breastfeeding, but there is no reliable way to verify what a child is being fed. As 'M'e Nthabiseng jokingly told me, "You can't always go there and squeeze milk out of them." Ultimately, women want what is best for their children, while simultaneously coping with competing sources of information, cultural expectations, intense social pressure, poverty, and hunger—all of which create magnified challenges for safe infant-feeding practices.

Monitoring the HIV status of exposed infants is also complex. In addition to the variety of ways infants can be exposed to HIV (during gestation, labor, and breastfeeding), the basic antibody test used on adults (the rapid test) does not accurately determine HIV status in children younger than 18 months because the mother's antibodies can persist in the child's blood until that time, resulting in a false positive. Therefore, children require a DNA/PCR blood test, which does not give immediate results, as the blood sample must be sent to the laboratory at the district hospital for analysis and the results sent back to the clinic. This process often takes several months. MCS outreach workers routinely checked their clients' health booklets (*bukana*) to ensure that a child's status was being properly monitored by the clinic or hospital. They often found that a child's test results had not been properly recorded in his or her health booklet. Confusion is compounded for orphans, as birth mothers are important sources of information when health-booklet records are incomplete.

Nondisclosure of HIV status is also a barrier for PMTCT. Effective PMTCT requires a woman to take several steps to protect her child. Many of these steps, such as exclusive breastfeeding and taking medication, are made easier by the support of family. Adherence is difficult if a woman has not disclosed her HIV status to those with whom she lives. One young woman I knew was pregnant with her third child, although one had been a stillbirth, and the other, a three-year-old, was HIV positive. She was living with her mother-in-law, to whom she had not disclosed her status. Because of this, she was unable to deliver at the hospital and did not receive the basic package to take at home, and the child became infected. Several months later, when I visited the family after the mother had disclosed her status, the grandmother repeated several times that she did not know the mother was supposed to go to the hospital, implying that she would have supported the mother if she had known. In this situation, the woman was attempting to balance a tenuous relationship with her mother-in-law and the health needs of her children.

'M'e Karabelo, an HIV-positive outreach worker, decided to test in 2005 after the devastating death of her four-month-old baby. In 2009, she married an HIV-positive man and told me that she wanted to have another child. She was hopeful that with the knowledge she had gained as an outreach worker—and since she had started ARVs—she would be able to prevent transmitting the virus to her child. In 2011, she gave birth to a beautiful baby boy, Limpho, who is now a healthy and HIV-free young child. For 'M'e Karabelo, PMTCT education was a key factor in avoiding the loss of another child. However, she was connected through her job to up-to-date and accurate information to which few other women have access. Women's participation in efforts to prevent mother-to-child transmission must be contextualized by the structural, cultural, and social factors that influence them. The very acts that are key to the process of establishing relatedness and nurturing life—sex, birth, breastfeeding, and caring—are also those that are responsible for the transmission of HIV. All these factors are complicated by the biocultural landscape in which they exist.

## TESTING KINSHIP

Across southern Africa, intervention efforts over the last decade have focused on the scale-up of HIV testing, since prevention and treatment for the disease, as well as funding, require baseline information that can be tricky to pin down: Who is seropositive? And how many are infected? While the mechanics of testing and the push to scale up are somewhat peripheral to the purview of kinship, HIV testing is central to the concerns of families and communities. First, it serves as the gateway to treatment, which, as I show further on, implicates kin in numerous ways. Second, in many cases, the intentionality around getting an HIV test implies both an admission of possible infection and the intent to act on information that could affect the health of one's sexual partners and children. Yet HIV testing is subject to its own set of challenges. Before the mid-2000s, in Lesotho, two faint pink lines on an HIV rapid test was a prediction of stigma, social ostracization, and certain death. People tried to hide their HIV status, even from families and sexual partners, until their physical symptoms betrayed them. Thankfully, this is no longer the case. As ARVs have become widely available, so have the people of Mokhotlong begun to queue in plain sight at clinics and hospitals, actively seeking to know their status. Yet although attitudes toward testing are increasingly positive, particular barriers limit its universal uptake, including gendered ideas about testing, ongoing stigma, and structural barriers such as limited access to VCT centers.

HIV testing in Lesotho is available in a variety of venues and is—at least in theory—voluntary. In 2014, almost all adults knew where to receive an HIV test, yet only 84 percent of women and 63 percent of men had ever been tested, and only 58 percent of women and 36 percent of men had been tested in the previous year (Lesotho Ministry of Health 2016). VCT counselors (like 'M'e Karabo) are trained and funded by a consortium of NGOs and work at hospitals, at clinics, and with organizations like New Start, who drive their mobile testing vans to towns, villages, and community gatherings. Every hospital and clinic has a designated VCT office where HIV testing and pre- and posttest counseling are done. VCT counselors also visit the inpatient wards at hospitals and do limited outreach and follow-up in rural areas.

By 2009, people from Mokhotlong's perceptions about HIV testing were generally positive, and many noted a marked improvement in public acceptance of testing. Most people I spoke with felt that an increasing number of Basotho were testing, and they often invoked the language of the government's national campaign, which encouraged everyone to "Know Your Status." Young 'M'e Matshepo's sentiments reflected this change: "People were encouraged to get tested and to know their status. But people refused to do that. Not like now, when they go to the clinic voluntarily." The pastor's wife, 'M'e Monatsi, agreed. "More people now are getting tested. They now have the courage," she said, referring to the growing acceptance of a potentially positive result. 'M'e Nthabiseng, trained in VCT, witnessed this normalization both among MCS clients and in the broader community: "Everyone that comes to us for support, and if we talk about HIV/AIDS testing, they are willing to test. . . . But the impact of the results, you can't see that much, because even if it's HIV/AIDS-positive, they still have babies. . . . But you can just see by looking outside Lerato Center, where they get HIV drugs and stuff, there are a ton of people every Monday and Wednesday to draw CD4—that's one of the signs that people are starting to act toward HIV and their own health." But as 'M'e Nthabiseng noted, people's willingness to test does not always result in changed behavior in terms of prevention, in part due to the continued importance of children.

Previously, people tested primarily when encouraged or coerced during interactions with health providers, such as during antenatal care or if hospitalized. However, other common routes to testing now exist. Some people simply decide that they would like to be tested and go to the clinic or hospital on their own. Others are encouraged by local support groups that go door to door. 'M'e Maliapeng said that she was encouraged to test by an HIV-positive friend who had noticed that she had lost weight. Many people who cared for an HIV-positive adult or child tested to ensure that they had not been infected while caregiving. The pastor and his wife, 'M'e and Ntate Monatsi, tested so that they could encourage their congregation to test without hypocrisy. 'M'e Monatsi noted, "If you want to talk to someone about it, having you yourself gone under it, knowing the experience of being there waiting for the results, how it feels. So then you can talk to other people about it." 'M'e Malefu told me that she went with other local village health workers for testing so that, like the Monatsis, they could lead by example.

Despite changing attitudes, persistent cultural ideals about masculinity discourage men from receiving medical treatment and voluntarily testing for HIV, particularly if they are still feeling healthy. As Mfecane (2012) notes, men's adherence to dominant norms of masculinity, including the desire for multiple partners and the lack of engagement with health care facilities, makes it difficult for them to act in the best interest of their own and their partners' health. Ntate Monatsi said, "Men are supposed to be strong and not just go [to the clinic] for each and every thing that is coming up." The outreach worker 'M'e Karabelo told me that men continue to be tested less because they rely on symptoms: "They believe that if you are going to the doctor, it's like you are weak. You have to be strong. You have to wait until it's bad, then you can come to the doctor." This reluctance to test was also tied to kinship; 'M'e Karabelo observed that men were afraid that a positive test would potentially reveal infidelity: "I don't know why. Maybe it's because they know that they are the one who is always coming out for, maybe for prostitution." 'M'e Masekha ventured that men were afraid of becoming overly medicalized. She told me, "They don't like it at all. Even when they are sick, and you encourage them to get tested, they will just go and consult the doctor and come back. . . . They are afraid. And they think when they get there, they will test positive, and they will go for the checkup every day." According to 'M'e Masekha, it was not just the results of the test that men feared but the actions that a positive test would require of them.

People with undiagnosed HIV often do not present with persistent symptoms until their viral load is high, which increases the risk of infecting sexual partners and lowers treatment success rates. 'M'e Mamohato's experience reinforces how men's reluctance to test has a negative impact on the physical and material health of the family and community and places particular strains on caregiving and kin relations. 'M'e Mamohato had two children and was pregnant with her third child when her husband, who had been feeling sick for many months, became increasingly ill and had to stop working. In addition to caring for her children, she was nursing her bedridden husband and trying to earn extra money for her family in secret, because her husband did not approve of her selling homemade brooms in town. She learned that she had HIV during antenatal care and encouraged her husband to test, but he refused, even though she disclosed her positive status to him. After several months, when he was already showing signs of the later stages of AIDS, he finally agreed to test, but he passed away before receiving treatment. 'M'e Mamohato noted a dramatic improvement in her own health after receiving treatment and lamented that perhaps her husband would have lived if he had agreed to test earlier. When I asked if she was angry with him, she laughed and told me, "There was no use being angry." Ntate Kapo, Kotsi's grandfather, told me in confidence that he was concerned about his brother, who was showing signs of infection. When I asked if he had encouraged his brother to test, he told me, "It's not something that he can do. Ah ah. I know him. I know how he is. . . . He's someone who doesn't listen to other people's encouragements." In both of these cases, family members seemed to accept men's distaste for medical interventions—particularly HIV tests—as inevitable, despite the high cost of remaining untested. When kin and familial bonds come into play, the implications of recommending an HIV test become increasingly fraught; 'M'e Mamohato waited until her husband was dying, and Ntate Kapo rejected the conversation with his brother altogether.

For the outreach worker 'M'e Karabelo, kinship and HIV testing intersected in a different way. Her husband's fear of testing and medical intervention led him to proclaim his positive status before it was even confirmed. 'M'e Karabelo, who had known her HIV status for several years, became engaged in 2009 after a brief courtship with a man she had known from childhood. Before she agreed to marry him, she told him of her status. At first, he was incredulous, asking her, "Are you lying to me?" She showed him her health booklet and medications as proof, which prompted him to reveal that he too was positive. But she was skeptical; when she asked to see his health booklet, he said that he had tested but had not received a CD4 count or any medications. Later, after a few months of marriage, he asked her if she wanted to have a baby. At this point, she insisted on having him tested to make sure his CD4 count was high in order to help prevent reinfection and mother-to-child transmission. He finally admitted that he had been lying—he didn't actually know his status; he'd never been tested. Perhaps he was trying to demonstrate that he still wanted to get married despite her status, or perhaps he suspected his status was positive. Either way, he preferred to lie about his status rather than actually submit to a test. When he finally did test, 'M'e Karabelo expressed relief at finally confirming his status. "I was worried about him," she told me, "because I see him. He is not healthy." After this, he initiated treatment, and she gave birth to a healthy baby boy.

Gender is not the only barrier to HIV testing. In the rural mountainous district of Mokhotlong, numerous social and structural barriers result in low testing rates, improper testing procedures, and increased stigma. In order to understand the testing experience, I went to the district hospital, located just down the road from MCS, to receive an HIV test myself. It took five trips to the hospital before I was able to obtain a test because I was unable to locate any of the counselors. The challenges I faced in obtaining an HIV test would likely be insurmountable for Basotho living in the outlying villages, who would need to overcome the inconvenience, cost, and fear of testing simply to arrive at the district hospital—let alone be turned away many times. Although these challenges were discouraging, they were not surprising. I was surprised, however, at how anxious I felt sitting in the waiting room and how my stomach churned while I waited for the little line to show up on the testing strip. This experience reinforced for me the importance of reducing barriers to test taking, including physical barriers, and the need for extensive VCT counselor training.

HIV-related stigma also discourages testing. Stigma is relevant only insofar as people fear its impact on their social relationships. In other words, stigma only exists in relation to other people. In a small, rural community such as

Mokhotlong, it would be nearly impossible for a Mosotho to go to their local health facility without encountering someone they knew. Many people said that they were not bothered by this, but some were reluctant to test for this reason. One young mother of an MCS client said that her friend did not test at the clinic because she thought that "people in the rural areas are silly," a term people use to refer to gossiping. Instead, she was tested by someone she knew who worked at a local NGO. For this same reason, 'M'e Nthabiseng offered HIV testing to the caregivers and family members of MCS clients and all MCS staff. One day, when I was in her office, she was setting up a testing kit. One of the house mothers came in with a baby, who I thought was getting tested. Instead, 'M'e Nthabiseng sent me out of the room with the baby in order to test the house mother. 'M'e Nthabiseng said that she sometimes wondered if MCS should offer HIV testing to the general public: "I kind of see people coming individually, feeling comfortable to come to MCS and get counseling and tested. So if we had an HIV counseling center, I think I have a strong belief that that would accommodate more people who would rather not go to the hospital but come here." However, when I asked her if this was in MCS's five-year plan, she keenly recognized that if MCS were to become a testing center, it would lose the exclusivity and sense of anonymity that currently makes it a comfortable place for clients and employees to get tested.

Testing is an important initial step in reducing the alarmingly high HIV rates in Lesotho, and thus efforts to reduce testing barriers are paramount. Like other intervention strategies for HIV, Mokhotlong residents' decisions to test or not are deeply influenced by their social networks, leaving people caught in a complex web of biocultural interactions. There is a dialectic relationship between testing and kinship, with testing decisions measured against their impact on kin, while kinship relationships influence both men's and women's testing decisions. These social factors are mediated by structural imbalances that unequally restrict Basotho's abilities to test, providing women with increased opportunities while reinforcing men's cultural proclivities against testing. As in all areas of HIV, these complex factors influence the most basic aspects of kinship and caregiving.

## TREATING HIV/AIDS

The provision and distribution of free antiretroviral drugs has been the single most important step toward a more effective response to HIV in southern Africa. Successful treatment affects the health of people living with HIV and their sexual partners and enables parents and caregivers to provide effective care to dependents. Once a patient overcomes the barriers leading to initiating HIV treatment, such as those that constrain him or her from testing, other challenges arise. Under ideal conditions, ART lessens a patient's viral load, reducing the chance of vertical (mother-to-child) and horizontal (usually sexual) transmission and increasing life expectancy. However, the sustained focus on biomedical intervention ignores the biocultural realties that will continue to limit the success of ART. In order to understand some of the challenges to successful HIV treatment in rural Lesotho, I conducted ethnographic observations at four different rural clinics in addition to my conversations with caregivers.

Mokhotlong residents who are educated about HIV treatment or who have seen the transformative power of treatment up close are more likely to have a positive view of ART. Many of the caregivers I spoke with had witnessed their children or grandchildren escape from the brink of death after receiving ARVs. Thapo's grandmother, for example, described her grandson's rapid recovery after starting ART: "*Kannete* (I swear), he was better after he started, and it was on the second month—2007. And on the fourth month, he gained weight, and he was a healthy child and living well. He has been healthy since that time. . . . He was sick. He was having diarrhea and vomiting, diarrhea and vomiting, and it is gone up to now."

'M'e Mamorena, who also saw the health of her granddaughter Hopolang dramatically improve with treatment, told me that people living with HIV should "run to the doctors" to stabilize the illness so that "it will not go anywhere." There are too many success stories like these to recount. Of course, the caregivers with whom I was acquainted were already positively predisposed to ART because their association with MCS implied a willingness to undergo testing and seek treatment when necessary, even if the motivation to do so was to receive MCS's services. If a client refuses to undergo HIV testing or repeatedly fails to adhere to a child's treatments, MCS reports the family to a social worker or the police and discontinues services to that family. MCS's limited support is only effective if caregivers fulfill their duties as treatment supporters; this means that occasionally, the most poorly cared-for children lose necessary support.

Poverty and food insecurity serve to exacerbate an already complex illness and put an almost unbearable burden on caregivers (Ncama et al. 2008; Bikaako-Kajura et al. 2006). Among pediatric patients at clinic visits, health care workers and caregivers frequently lamented food shortages and malnutrition. According to the most recent demographic health survey, nearly half of children under five in Mokhotlong had stunting, which is a sign of chronic undernutrition, and 16 percent of children had moderate to severe malnutrition (Lesotho Ministry of Health 2016). Furthermore, food insecurity has worsened with lower agricultural yields due to droughts, soil erosion, and overgrazing, and families have reduced access to cash remittances (Himmelgreen et al. 2009; Leduka et al. 2015). A starch-heavy diet of maize meal (*papa*) and porridge (*lesheleshele*) is sorely lacking in nutrients and protein, particularly in winter, when leafy greens are sparse. Additionally, children with undiagnosed HIV or TB (tuberculosis) often have suppressed appetites and may fail to thrive regardless of what they are fed. For this reason, MCS's nutritional assistance consists mainly of milk or formula and protein in the form of soy, beans, peas, and canned fish. Some MCS clients also receive chickens in order to have a steady source of eggs. If malnutrition is severe, ideally it is treated with a ready-to-use therapeutic food (RUTF) such as Plumpy Nut, a pouch of peanut butter–like paste that contains all the necessary fats, proteins, and nutrients for weight gain. But it can be difficult to get children to eat the recommended amount, which they are supposed to finish before they have any other food for the day. Field notes from my clinic observations highlight the multiple challenges of poverty and malnutrition for a 17-month-old child, HIV positive but not yet on ART:

> This child has been vomiting for two weeks every day after taking medication. Has very bad sores in the mouth. Not on ARVs. Child not breastfeeding or eating. The child is stage 4 because she is severely malnourished and has thrush and herpes. The child needs ARVs soon. The nurse tried giving her Plumpy Nut to see if she would eat it but she cannot eat it probably because of the sores in her mouth. Child is referred to the hospital. During the clinic visit the mother was crying and said it was because they have no money for the hospital.

In this case, the child was suffering from poverty, severe illness, and multiple serious opportunistic infections. These kinds of complicated and multilayered cases are common and difficult to address.

The moral stakes of supporting a child living with HIV are high because survival depends on good adherence and medical compliance by someone else on his or her behalf. In my clinical observations, only two out of 42 children were not accompanied by a caregiver. In one case, a 17-year-old girl came in with her own baby, and in the other, a teenage girl came alone because her usual treatment supporter, her grandmother, was sick. However, for complicated drug regimens, a consistent caregiver is extremely important, and in my clinic observations, a change in caregivers frequently led to poor adherence among children. Additionally, some children seemed to be in the care of a reluctant relative, and therefore, the quality of care they received was inadequate. One 13-year-old girl, who contracted HIV as an infant, came in on two separate occasions with her aunt, who was her primary caregiver. My field notes state, "Patient has been on ARVs for over two years. She was doing poorly a month ago. Dr. N is worried she is failing her first-line treatment. May need second-line but that is difficult to get. Also, need to be sure she can have good adherence before switching. Coughing especially when sleeping. The child looks very sick and is extremely wasted. She looks about eight years old. Her adherence is also very poor (93 percent, 57 percent, 83 percent). The aunt denies failing to give her any meds even though it is obvious that she has been missing them." I later learned that the patient passed away six months after this visit, reinforcing how essential it is to have willing and informed caregivers. Even if second-line ARVs had been approved, it is unlikely that her adherence or her social supports would have improved, abandoning her to the same fate.

The painful way in which HIV flows through families was exhibited during one clinic visit. A 42-year-old man came in to the clinic with his 40-year-old wife and 20-month-old child. The wife did not appear to understand why they were at the clinic, and it was eventually revealed that the husband, who had been on ART for several months, had not disclosed his status to his wife. Obviously nervous, he brought her to the appointment as a way of informing her of his status so that she could get tested. The man had poor adherence, likely because he had not disclosed his status to his wife and was forced to take his medication in secret and without support. The man went home after his visit, and the wife and child went to the counseling center next door, where a government-trained counselor is required to perform the test and provide comprehensive pre- and posttest counseling. When the woman and child returned to the nurse's office, clutching referrals for a blood draw, it was obvious from the mother's face that the news was not good; both tests had been positive. The nurse asked if the counselor had informed her about what her diagnosis meant and what next steps she must take; she replied that the counselor had merely performed the test and left. It was late in the day, and it is likely the counselor wanted to go home, so she skipped the required posttest counseling. The mother returned to the nurse's office scared and visibly shaken, her sickly baby crying in her arms. While the way in which the man disclosed his status to his wife perhaps displays a lack of marital communication, at least he was there. There are many who never come.

On my most recent trip to Lesotho, in 2015, I became concerned that Tsepi, then 11 years old, was failing his first-line ARVs. He had been on the treatment since 2006 and had excellent adherence but had developed a persistent rash on his body and visible painful growths in both his eyes that caused him to squint in the sun, though he was always smiling in his good-natured way. I brought him to the district hospital and also had him follow-up with a Ugandan doctor, Dr. Gillian, who worked for an American university hospital that runs a pediatric AIDS clinic in Mokhotlong. It took several months to get Tsepi's viral load because his sample had to be processed at the lab in Maseru. These lab results were then sent to an advisory board along with a letter written by Dr. Gillian proving that, despite good adherence, his viral load was low—a sign of treatment failure. After many months, his second-line treatment was approved. Tsepi's caregivers would have never been able to advocate for him without external help. It took several extra trips to his village and the clinic and hospital, and transportation money for those trips was beyond their means. Furthermore, neither his family nor the rural nurses were trained or equipped at that time to recognize possible treatment failure. It was mostly because of the hard work and advocacy of Dr. Gillian (and his luck both at being connected to this *lekhooa* and that his treatment failure became evident during one of my trips) that Tsepi is now on second-line ARVs. But this haphazard approach is not a sustainable way for residents of Mokhotlong to gain access to lifesaving treatment. It is a vital and largely unrecognized issue that many people will experience treatment failure before it is widely recognized by health care providers in Lesotho. At that point, the legal battle to receive generic second-line drugs will need to be waged, as it was for first-line drugs in South Africa in 2001 (Sidley 2001). I continue to hope that my friends and interlocutors will be behind this curve rather than in front of it.

## "AN ILLNESS JUST LIKE ANYTHING ELSE": SIGNS OF STIGMA REDUCTION

Families in the highlands of Lesotho have been living with HIV for over a quarter of a century, yet residents of Mokhotlong still hesitate when discussing the illness that has cruelly infected their families and their lives. Instead of calling HIV by its name, many people refer to it as "that disease" or, starkly, "it." One grandmother referred to it as "the illness of *H*," while another called it "the disease for the youth." Even 'M'e Maliapeng, who told me unprompted about her status, still denied initially that her husband died of HIV, saying it was TB and only later admitting that he had tested positive. Others, when asked about a loved one's illness, would focus on the symptoms of the patient in question rather than actually identifying HIV as the problem. HIV is seldom written on death certificates or openly acknowledged as the cause of death by family members and friends at funerals. Yet despite these outward signs of ongoing stigma, even in the short decade of my research in Mokhotlong, things have gotten better.

Stigma surrounding HIV has been well documented across southern Africa (Skinner and Mfecane 2004; Holzemer et al. 2007; Kalichman and Simbayi 2003; Mahajan et al. 2008). It is pervasive and persists across all aspects of HIV management, from caregiving to treatment. Stigma does not have meaning outside of its social context. The mere existence of stigma is evidence of the intersection between HIV and kinship because stigma, at its core, is the fear of negative social ramifications and their impact on networks of kin and care. One of the most promising signs of stigma reduction for HIV in Mokhotlong is implied by local characterizations of the illness. Prior to the mid-2000s, HIV was a swift and highly visible killer. Since then, the availability of treatment has allowed Basotho living with HIV to lead relatively healthy and stable lives for many years. As Ntate Kanelo noted, people still talk about HIV, but the tenor of their conversations has changed because "there is something helping people to get better. There were many people dying in the past." Because of this, many people in Mokhotlong, such as Tsepiso's mother, explained to me that HIV was "an illness just like anything else." 'M'e Nthabiseng expressed these same sentiments about her foster daughter, Lerato, by calling her illness "normal." This attitude was common among patients and caregivers and is an important sign not only of stigma reduction but of coping mechanisms that help people "live positively" (a common slogan, globally, encouraging safe sex, good adherence, and stigma reduction).

Another important sign of stigma reduction takes shape in the increased communication about HIV between kin. Only a few years ago, many elderly residents of Mokhotlong reported to me that they did not know the cause of death of the adult children who had died in their arms. Prior to the availability of ART, there was little incentive to be tested or disclose. Finally, after decades of living with AIDS and over a decade into available treatment, the lines of communication have opened. According to the VCT counselor 'M'e Karabo, couples are increasingly being tested together. In contrast to those caregivers whose children died of unknown causes, many caregivers have now helped support loved ones in adhering to complex treatment regimens.

Many couples, such as the Ntho family (Matseli's grandparents), told me that they encouraged each other to test and went to the counseling center together. During one visit to their village, 'M'e Ntho and I were sitting at her kitchen table in her rondavel discussing HIV-prevention strategies when Ntate Ntho returned home from the fields. I paused and asked if they were comfortable continuing the conversation together given the sensitive topic, and they both agreed that it was fine. In contrast, on a previous occasion, Ntate Ntho entered the home while I was discussing issues surrounding birthing practices with 'M'e Ntho, and both husband and wife thought it better to discuss such things separately. On a visit to 'M'e Maphonolo with the MCS outreach team, she told me that she was comfortable with her friend remaining in her home while MCS was counseling her on PMTCT because, she said, "she is someone I trust. I have seen that she doesn't care. There is nothing that she will not do with me." I also discussed HIV and marriage with 'M'e Masenate, the young caregiver of Tebello, and her neighbor 'M'e Matsiu. I was surprised to find out that these two young women, who spent much time together and spoke easily with me about HIV, had never previously discussed the matter with each other. People's openness to engage in conversations about HIV and their apparent comfort level during our discussions signaled a desire to find safe venues for dialogue. This need for facilitated conversations about HIV was reinforced when, near the end of my fieldwork, several caregivers thanked me for speaking with them. 'M'e Malefu, the village health worker and caregiver, said, "Thank you, because you have made me to be wise about things I wasn't aware of." 'M'e Mapole, the caregiver for chronically

ill Letlo, thanked me "because when we are talking, it is like you are also counseling me." There is evidently a latent willingness to talk about HIV that could
be harnessed if the proper format for conversations was fostered. While such
conversations may not occur spontaneously, making space for them could be an
important step toward stigma reduction and AIDS education.

One potential venue for facilitating such conversations could be through
patient support groups where patient supporters (*batsihetsi*) provide physical,
emotional, and material support for people living with HIV/AIDS. Several of the
grandmothers with whom I spoke were members of such support groups, which
are usually organized at the village or community level by chiefs or through
church groups. Women often bring soap, do laundry, or help cook and bathe
patients, often in the late stages of AIDS, when these daily tasks become difficult. They also keep fairly accurate records—usually handwritten in old school
notebooks—of all the orphaned and vulnerable children in the village, whom
they helped me locate many times throughout the years, often accompanying
me from house to house. Although increasing communication about HIV/
AIDS is not currently central to these groups' mission, there is the potential to
utilize these established forums to foster improved AIDS education and reduce
the sources of gossip and hearsay that hinder prevention and treatment efforts.

Stigma reduction was also signaled by everyday interactions between people.
Prior to the widespread availability of ARVs, fear and misinformation ostracized
people living with AIDS. In a 2004 South African study, 26 percent of respon-
dents said that they would not be willing to share a meal, 18 percent would not
sleep in the same room, and 6 percent would not speak with a person they knew
to be HIV positive (Kalichman and Simbayi 2004). However, this appears to
be no longer the case, at least in Mokhotlong. 'M'e Maphonolo said that in the
past, people did not want to share things like *joala* (home-brewed beer) and porridge because it required eating from the same basin. Shared food is an important
mechanism for creating and maintaining social relationships, and the refusal to
share food can be a powerful tool in weakening social networks. Although she
admitted that while some people still do not want to share, most people are comfortable sharing food, even if they are aware of someone's HIV-positive status.
She told me, "They know that they will not infect them. They can only be infected
by blood. You cannot be infected by saliva. I have seen other people not caring
because they say it's the disease all over the world, and how will people know that
they will not suffer from it?" As she implies, the pervasiveness of HIV in Lesotho
has resulted in stigma reduction, perhaps because interacting with HIV-positive
people is unavoidable or perhaps because increased interaction with HIV-
positive people helps reduce fear and increase knowledge about likely modes of
transmission. Despite these encouraging signs, stigma remains a barrier for interventions targeting all areas of HIV prevention, testing, and treatment in Lesotho.

## CONCLUSION: PRIVILEGING KINSHIP

AIDS has made its way into every Mosotho family. Ntate Kapo, whose grandson is infected and who lost his daughter, his brother, his sister-in-law, and eventually his own life to HIV, told me simply, "It makes Basotho suffer." The root causes of this suffering are not poor medical adherence, promiscuity, or misguided cultural beliefs about prevention and treatment strategies—the root causes are poverty and inequality. Global political-economic structures have become naturalized in a way that leads people to think it unfair but inevitable that an American can access virtually limitless treatment for AIDS at insignificant cost, while a Mosotho in Mokhotlong can access only one course of treatment—perhaps two if lucky and well connected. These unequal structures—comprising poor and failing health systems, understaffed hospitals and clinics, inefficient supply chains, and poor transportation—are violent in the way they make it permissible to value some lives over others. While structural violence can be measured by looking at the unequal distribution of disease through human populations, it most powerfully manifests in the everyday lives of families and communities. When Ntate Kalasi, the HIV-positive and disabled father of five, once asked me if I thought a cure for the disease was possible, I told him, perhaps naively, that I did think so and that many doctors were working on it. Ntate Kalasi looked at me for a moment before responding. "But all people will be dead," he said. "They will all be gone."

The ethnographic examples that I have detailed here illuminate the often fuzzy connections between everyday experiences and broader structural processes. In making these connections with the continued spread of HIV in Lesotho, this work confirms the multiple intersections between HIV and kinship. Many of the examples implicate kin and care in both direct and indirect ways. In deciding about prevention, testing, and treatment, patients and caregivers grapple with competing messages and pervasive (if declining) stigma. Within this context, caregivers conduct daily negotiations about the costs and benefits of their actions on the health of children in their care and on their broader social networks.

By understanding how HIV impacts the social fabric of everyday life, we can see how it has fundamentally changed the structure and role of caregiving relationships in Lesotho. The following chapter will examine how HIV has altered the organization and makeup of the family by focusing on the important role of the caregiver while moving away from idealized notions of patrilineality. However, the ways in which Basotho negotiate for the care of orphans still exists firmly within the familiar tropes of lineal ideals, even as caregiving practices emerge as increasingly flexible and central to Basotho notions of kinship.

# 4 · ORPHAN CARE
# AND THE FAMILY

## The Labor and Love of 'M'e Matau

*Five dust balls blew across the earthen floor of 'M'e Matau's rondavel before reveal-
ing themselves to be tiny gray chicks, meager sprites that skittered around the room
and then huddled behind a hand-cranked maize mill, a heavy cast-iron thing sitting in
the shadows by the wall. The chicks' mother advanced, squawking, toward Ellen, then
snagged awkwardly: her left spur was bound to the maize mill with a strip of cloth.*

*It was a glorious day in February, and in the cool of the rondavel, Ellen and
'M'e Matau had been talking about love or lust or marital things even more
complicated—the kinds of things one discusses on hot summer days when provided
refuge from the sun. Back then, 'M'e Matau was 55 or 69; it wasn't entirely clear.
Nkhono had supplied Ellen with two possible birth years but couldn't settle on one.
"Maybe 1945?" she suggested, providing a third option, just to be safe.*

*Anyway, it didn't really matter. Ellen had traveled to 'M'e Matau's rondavel to hear
the story of how she came to marry her husband.*

*"He was just some boy," nkhono said, laughing. "I didn't know him."*

*This caught Ellen up. "Are you saying he stole you?" she asked, referring to the prac-
tice called* chobeliso, *outlawed now by the government although still fresh in cultural
memory—still practiced infrequently and discreetly in rural Lesotho.*

*"Ache, no, he didn't steal me. He liked my family. The boy just came to me and said
he wanted to fall in love with me. I told him to talk to my parents."*

*And so it blossomed, back in 19xx (Ellen had stopped pressing for her birth year
by this point), back when the boy's parents had struck a deal with her own parents:
"There was no white wedding, it just went like that. His parents came to collect me,
and they paid* likhomo—*ten cows."*

*"We fell in love," nkhono said and paused, looking out into the blinding day. Her
husband had been dead for just over a year now.*

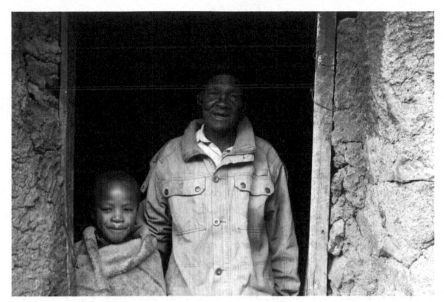

FIGURE 4.1. 'M'e Matau and her grandson, Tsepi, stand in the doorway to their home, Mokhotlong, 2015

*"In the old days, things were better," she continued, drawing on that line of reasoning we all must pursue after a certain age, regardless of gender or geography. "In those days, people were happier. A wife might get upset if the husband was always going to parties and playing his accordion late—but they would still be happy. . . . When we fought, I would go back to my home, and he would come to collect me . . . so we stopped fighting. Kannete, we were happy."*

*Ellen asked her what things were like now, how times had changed.*

*"People now are just getting divorced. They say they will pay* likhomo*, but they don't. So when they fight, the wife leaves and knows she can find another husband."*

*Over by the maize mill, the mother hen had hunkered down in front of her chicks, murmuring protectively and eyeing Ellen with a measure of avian coolness. The rondavel was immaculate—the floor swept and the tiny space in meticulous order. Outside, a deep-ribbed dog lay sleeping in the shade of the thatched overhang.*

*"Everything about the way we are living has changed," 'M'e Matau said. "The earth has changed. I see women wearing trousers now, wearing caps made for men."*

*For 'M'e Matau, things have changed most noticeably in her daily caregiving. For the last several years,* nkhono *has been raising three grandchildren, the children of her daughters. One of these daughters died in 2006, and while MCS's (Mokhotlong Children's Services) records indicate that the woman was HIV positive, 'M'e Matau has a different understanding of her daughter's death.*

"She was sick with high blood and painful feet," she told Ellen. "The high blood came from her work, where there was money missing. The owner was thinking the laborers had stolen it, but it was the owner's own child who did it." This stressful work environment, this false accusation of theft—'M'e Matau believed—led to her daughter's illness.

This daughter had left behind three children; Tsepi, the youngest, is also HIV positive. The boy was six months old and very sick when his mother died. But 'M'e Matau brought him to MCS, where he lived for nine months. Tsepi is healthy now, has been on meds for years, and has grown into a sturdy child, nearly four years old.

As 'M'e Matau and Ellen talked in the rondavel, Tsepi ran in to complain to his grandmother, out of breath and aggrieved that his cousins were harassing him. Nkhono told the boy to leave so she could talk with her guest, telling him to wipe his nose as he went, and Tsepi turned, slump-shouldered, and drifted back into the day. Ellen had met him several times before. Whenever 'M'e Matau came into town, she made a point of visiting the safe home to say hello, each time accompanied by Tsepi, dressed in his finest: denim head to toe, with a patchwork jacket and matching jeans.

It was a world in flux that 'M'e Matau depicted for Ellen that day. There were four grandchildren, nkhono said, but then one died. Tsepi's mother was married, nkhono said, but then she divorced, and then she died. The grandchildren all stayed in her house, nkhono said, unless the older kids stayed with other relatives closer to their school. Everything was fluid, everything in circulation.

Ellen heard a cry and looked out into the sunlight. Tsepi ran past the doorway then, in hot pursuit of his cousins with a shovelful of rocks, his four-year-old body chugging away earnestly, belting gleeful war cries all the way.

* * *

During the harvest, Ellen found 'M'e Matau working in a neighbor's field. Nkhono's sweater was covered entirely in burrs that day, a layer of golden fur. The two walked to the side of the road, where they could sit and talk in the sun, looking out across fields that descended from the road in a shallow bowl. The terraced fields were lined like sheet music, and piles of maize stalks sat at irregular intervals along those lines—quarter notes in an unplayable score, some pastoral symphony written for the hawks and other coasting raptors.

Ellen had come with a knit hat for Tsepi, anticipating the coming winter. As she received the gift, 'M'e Matau told Ellen how much Tsepi loved bragging about these small tokens. Just yesterday, he had run through the rondavel, brandishing a tiny package and calling out to his cousins, "This is the soap my lekhooa gave me!"

Nkhono's life caring for Tsepi and the other children had continued apace since Ellen's last visit. And while challenging, it was certainly a familiar experience for 'M'e Matau. As a girl, she had lived with her own nkhono, an arrangement between her parents and her grandmother. "They liked me to stay with her to fetch some water," 'M'e Matau said. Even though her parents lived in another corner of the same village, 'M'e Matau spent her early childhood through age 15 sleeping and eating in her grandmother's rondavel. It was there that she helped with daily chores, things like collecting firewood and doing the wash.

"I liked it so much," 'M'e Matau said. "She taught me stories and riddles—and when I went to school, I was telling the other children what I had learned from my grandmother." It was in her grandmother's house, for instance, that 'M'e Matau learned the riddle of Masilo and Masilonyane: Masilo of my mother and Masilo of my mother—but you know that one. It was an old joke even when 'M'e Matau was a girl.

Child fostering like this was common in Lesotho even before AIDS burned through the countryside and forced families to adapt their ideas of caregiving. Children left their parents and lived with relatives for any number of reasons—from educational opportunities to apprenticeships to various familial obligations. "Kannete, it is good," 'M'e Matau told Ellen, referring to Basotho child-fostering practices. "It is good for both the child and the grandparent."

Tsepi's paternal grandparents seemed to think so too. After Tsepi's mother died in 2006, the parents of Tsepi's dead father made a claim on the boy and his siblings. They didn't talk with 'M'e Matau directly—who had been caring for her dying daughter in addition to the children—but instead sent her a letter. They would not lose their babies, it said. The grandchildren were theirs.

Perhaps driven by the businesslike mode of their request, 'M'e Matau laid out a legalistic rebuttal. "I didn't agree with them," she told Ellen. "They hadn't taken responsibility before." She said that side of the family had never housed the children properly, and Tsepi's father hadn't taken care of their mother. This was all important, but the legal crux of her argument hinged on the likhomo: those people had never paid it, only agreed on a number, and so they had no true claim on the children.

"They never sent cows," 'M'e Matau said and sat back, satisfied that she had demonstrated her case. Across the fields, the sun had ignited the clouds in slow motion, the horizon ablaze with gaudy pinks and oranges.

"Why do you think the other grandparents wanted Tsepi and his siblings?" Ellen asked.

"They just want these children to work for them," 'M'e Matau said.

"And why did you want to keep them?"

"I like them to help me too—because I have been caring for them."

\* \* \*

The years rolled along, as years are entitled to do. On a trip back to Lesotho in 2013, Ellen trekked out to 'M'e Matau's village one day, where she found that word of her *visit had slightly preceded her. Children had seen Ellen on the hillside and scrambled ahead. Now a crowd was gathering before 'M'e Matau's rondavel, curious neighbors and schoolchildren detoured from their usual routes home.*

*People were pleased to see Ellen again, but it was Eve—our one-year-old, strapped to Ellen's back and moderately perturbed at the fuss—who quickly became a celebratory focal point. 'M'e Matau rushed off to find an appropriate welcoming gift and returned with an equally perturbed and thoroughly ruffled chicken for Eve, a bird of mottled black-and-white feathers whom we later named 'M'e Macaroni. She was perhaps the adult incarnation of one of those five dust balls from a few years back—although who could say where the wind had circulated those chicks in the meantime.*

*Twenty people crowded into 'M'e Matau's rondavel to observe while Ellen and nkhono caught up on the intervening years. There was a general sense of relief at the news that Ellen had given birth to two children since her last visit. Her previous status as a married woman of childbearing age—and yet childless—had troubled many people. Since child fostering was so common, people had initially assumed that Ellen had children living with relatives somewhere else and were unsettled to discover that they simply did not exist.*

*But that matter was put to rest now. As 'M'e Matau continued to note, everything was fluid, everything in circulation. Some of the children she had been caring for had gone on to live with other relatives in other places. Tsepi was still living with her, a happy seven-year-old with a gap in his smile from recently vacated milk teeth.*

*"He is doing well," 'M'e Matau said. "You can see that he is well."*

*For a moment, though, she was back somewhere perilous in 2006. "You know, I didn't believe that he would live—"*

*But her reminiscence was cut short by Eve: the girl had been on an exploratory crawl around the rondavel, and 'M'e Matau leaned over to stop her from eating a handful of ashes.*

*"He is well," 'M'e Matau said again, looking over at Tsepi. "The boy is healthy."*

*Recently, though, she had begun making arrangements for what would happen to Tsepi after her death, something that caregivers usually leave for their surviving relatives to sort out at the funeral. Nkhono wanted to make sure that someone in the family would care for him after she was gone. Death had been on her mind lately. She told Ellen that death was changing the Basotho family—and not just the deaths of older people like her but the deaths caused by that disease for the youth. It was important, then, to make sure there were people in the extended family who could care for orphaned children.*

*Ellen asked her why this was so important. Why—with all the challenges that came from taking on another dependent, whether financial or physical or emotional—why was it better for a child to avoid the orphanage?*

*'M'e Matau couldn't conceive of another way. She said it was necessary for an orphaned child to stay with relatives, even if it meant the child had to move from place to place occasionally.*

*"It would make him forget that he is an orphan," she said, and people in the ron-davel murmured their assent. "He can grow up and know that he still has his family."*

-WM-

\* \* \*

## NEGOTIATING CARE

Like many of the grandmothers I spoke with, 'M'e Matau lived with her own maternal grandmother from early childhood until she was 15 years old—even though she was only a short walk from the house where her parents and siblings lived—sent to provide companionship and to assist her grandmother with household chores. Now grandmothers like 'M'e Matau (and a small but growing number of grandfathers) use what they know from their own fostering experiences to accommodate the shifting domestic arrangements that stem from increasing numbers of orphans. While this recent increase is perhaps more dramatic due to the severity and scale of AIDS, caregiving practices like child fostering have always been in flux, responding to historical and political-economic circumstances. Idealized norms are seldom closely followed in practice, yet the persistence of these ideals and the different ways they are *not* followed continue to be illuminating.

In Lesotho, child fostering has a long history as a strategy for sharing responsibility and supporting and connecting kin (Page 1989; Murray 1981). Unsurprisingly, however, fostering practices in Lesotho have had to adapt to the demographic pressures of HIV/AIDS. AIDS mortality and the large orphan population have altered the makeup of households and reinforced the importance of cohabitation in shaping relatedness. Families appear to be adapting by capitalizing on the flexibility and fluidity of household membership and the normalcy of child circulation in order to understand this new order within the context of the old rules. Even though 'M'e Matau was a maternal relative, she used the rules of patrilineal descent and the importance of bridewealth payments to justify her claim to her grandchildren. This kind of reinterpretation of social practices is slowly changing the makeup of families in Mokhotlong, resulting in a system of caregiving that is increasingly flexible: care arrangements can remain within the ideal of patrilineality while finding another shape entirely. In many ways, care for orphans is similar to the care that nonorphaned children in Mokhotlong receive. Thus, as Henderson warns (2011), the popular imaginaries that circulate about orphans as destitute and outside the moral reach of the family are largely untrue. But orphanhood is a permanent condition (as opposed to child circulation for purposes of companionship or assistance) that produces a unique set of social and economic challenges.

There has been a gradual shift among Basotho families toward increasing care by maternal relatives, the majority being grandmothers. While the process of negotiation and justification that occurs when families are deciding on the locality of care for orphans remains couched in terms of patrilineal descent, the affective elements of care—that is, who is most willing and able to provide the daily labor of caregiving—have emerged as the strongest motivators for new patterns of social organization. This general trend that places women at the heart of many Basotho families—what Cecile Jackson (2015) calls the "matrifocal turn"—is characteristic of contemporary forms of relatedness and can sit comfortably alongside any system of lineality.

Bourdieu's differentiation (1977) between "official" and "practical" kin helps explain the gap between kinship ideologies and caring practices for Basotho. Where "official kin" is the representation of kinship for the public sphere by the group as a whole, "practical kin" is "directed toward the satisfaction of the practical interests of an individual or group of individuals" (1977, 35). People actively forge relationships based on their practical needs, in spite of the tenets of "official kin" doctrine. As Sherry Ortner argues, even though culture "shapes, guides, and even to some extent dictates behavior" (1984, 152), rules have never merely been followed. While Basotho may frame their negotiations as structured by an inflexible set of rules, they work within a series of competing ideologies—or as Comaroff puts it, a "repertoire of potential manipulations" (1978, 4).

Kinship continues to be intrinsic to the very notion of care; consequently, few orphans are cared for outside the fold of family. Increasingly, the willingness to provide care, or what Borneman calls "processes of voluntary affiliation" (1997, 574), as demonstrated by everyday acts of caring, have become most important in influencing patterns of child circulation. This, in turn, impacts the very nature of relationships between kin (Klaits 2010). The emergence and uncertainty of matrilocal care must be understood as embedded in a context that is constrained not only by AIDS and poverty but by historical and political-economic shifts—such as migrant labor and apartheid—that span over a century. While these structural changes are still being understood within the patrilineal context, I suspect that there will be a normative shift away from the current ideal of patrilineality—at least when it comes to caregiving. The beginning of this shift is evident in the negotiations, justifications, and practices that caregivers employ in Mokhotlong. At the local level, the experiences of the caregivers who fill these pages provide a greater understanding of the changes within families and households in rural Lesotho because of HIV. At a broader level, this exploration provides insight into the ways that kinship structures change incrementally and over time due to major social disruption. As exceptional behavior is normalized, conceptions about what is considered ideal change, lessening the gap between the ideal and practice.

In this chapter, I begin by examining the physical components of care—from the fluidity and movement of children in and out of households to the day-to-day challenges of caregiving—in the context of the Basotho history of child-fostering practices. This examination of past and current fostering practices highlights local perceptions of "good" care and the important relationship between the elderly and the young, especially between children and their grandmothers. I then turn to the challenges unique to caring for children living with HIV, who are frequently orphaned at the height of their illness and whose ongoing medical needs are numerous. Finally, I turn my attention to the theoretical crux of this work: the shift toward matrilocal care in the context of strongly idealized patrilineal norms and the negotiations that reflect new practices while reifying firmly entrenched ideals.

## CHILD FOSTERING, INTERGENERATIONAL AFFECTION, AND "GOOD" CAREGIVERS

The normalcy and frequency of child fostering in rural households in Mokhotlong is immediately apparent. Throughout childhood, children regularly live with various relatives on both the paternal and maternal sides. Many parents in Lesotho leave their children with relatives while they work in the lowlands of Lesotho or in South Africa (Lesotho Bureau of Statistics 2008). Informal child fostering based on kin relations is common and has been studied extensively, including in sub-Saharan Africa (Bledsoe 1990; Renne 1993; Goody 1984; Isiugo-Abanihe 1985), Oceania (Carroll 1970; Carsten 1991), Latin America (Leinaweaver 2008; Fonesca 2004; Walmsley 2008), and in marginalized communities in the United States, where it is typically called "kinship care" (Grant 2000; Crumbley and Little 1997). Child fostering may benefit children and their parents by reducing the economic burden on the family, giving the child improved educational opportunities, providing the child with vocational training or an apprenticeship, helping wean a child in order to increase fertility, or simply establishing social ties that will benefit the child and family in the future (Renne 1993; Bledsoe 1989; Goody 1984). Child fostering also benefits the caregivers by providing companionship, daily assistance, and economic security (Bledsoe 1989).

Despite numerous characterizations of fostering as fundamentally reciprocal (Bledsoe 1989), such practices are not always beneficial or voluntary. Several scholars have highlighted the role of poverty in the circulation of children, often transferring the productive contributions of children from one household to another (Leinaweaver 2007; Schrauwers 1999; Goody 1982). In a review of kin-based informal fostering practices around the world, Jessaca Leinaweaver teased out the types of fostering relationships that were beneficial to children and those that were not. She found that when fostering expands the family rather than limits it, involves input from the child in question, or is purposefully targeting educational or employment opportunities, it typically advances a child's economic and social well-being. When the movement of children is a response to hardship—poverty, inequality, or disease, for instance—it can negatively affect children's attachments, lead to the differential treatment of children in a new household, and take advantage of socioeconomic disparities by exploiting their labor (Leinaweaver 2014). Fostering practices in Lesotho are not straightforward or unambiguously positive. Yet while they frequently emerge in response to a crisis in care and are often accompanied by complex health needs, they are still viewed as mutually beneficial and as positive kin-strengthening strategies.

African scholarship has documented the many ways that children contribute to fostering households (Renne 1993; Bledsoe 1989; Goody 1984; Page 1989). In Lesotho, children are expected to perform a number of chores, including cooking, laundry, collecting wood, collecting water, helping in the fields, and tending to animals. As Bray (2003) notes, defining housework in a southern African context as child labor does not take into account the cultural view of this type of work as an essential part of household membership and social learning. Although some fostering relationships are ethically ambiguous in terms of the balance between labor and care, most adults in rural Lesotho remember their childhood fostering experiences as overwhelmingly positive, even if they were expected to perform regular household and agricultural duties. Basotho children also enjoy a great deal of leisure time. Although many caregivers spoke about the assistance that their foster children provided, I more often than not observed children playing with their friends rather than working. Caregivers, on the other hand, were usually hard at work whenever I dropped by their homes. Zimmerman and her colleagues define carework as "the multifaceted labor that produces the daily living conditions that make basic human health and well-being possible" (2006, 3). The authors specifically include human health in order to capture the nursing, nurturing, and caring tasks common to many women globally. As in many other places, this day-to-day caregiving in Lesotho remains primarily in the female domain (Robson et al. 2006). Thus the caregivers I worked with were mostly women, and the ethnographic examples reflect this reality.

The widespread fostering practices that have helped many orphaned Basotho children find homes within their extended networks of kin are not new. Current fostering practices are part of a long tradition that many caregivers experienced as children themselves. One major factor that facilitates the care of children within the family network is the strong bond between alternate generations, a longstanding trope in anthropology (Lévi-Strauss 1969; Radcliffe-Brown and Forde 1951). As Alber (2004) notes for Benin, the elderly view the process as a circular exchange that benefits individuals both at the beginning and end of their lives. Children in Mokhotlong often go to live with relatives when their mothers are trying to wean them and sometimes stay for years. More than half of the caregivers I got to know well spoke about living for an extended period with other relatives when they were young, usually maternal or paternal grandmothers but a few with aunts or with both of their grandparents. In all of these cases, only one could be considered crisis fostering (due to a mother's death), with one other due to a mother's migration for work. The rest lived with relatives for mutually beneficial reasons including companionship, love and affection, and assistance. Sometimes the children would relocate with a sibling or cousin, and sometimes they would go by themselves. When I asked 'M'e Mapole why she went to live with her grandmother as a child, she told me, "She didn't have any children living with her. And my mother said she should take care of me so that I could help her when I grew up." 'M'e Mapole's mother explicitly sought to create a bond of affection and mutual assistance between grandmother and granddaughter. Most of my interlocutors, like 'M'e Mapole, had fond memories of living with their grandmothers. "My grandmother loved me, and I loved her too," 'M'e Mapoloko said. "[Grandmothers] were taking good care of the children because they loved them. They were asking a girl, 'What do you need?'"

Although household work was expected of children, if a child was required to do too much work or if a caregiver was perceived as lazy, others in the community would be highly critical. 'M'e Marefiloe, who provided well for her great-granddaughter, Nkhabu, was critical of the girl's paternal grandmother, who cared for Nkhabu's two brothers. "Those boys are gathering wood," she told me, "and the grandmother is not doing that. She would rather take the roof off her house to make a fire, and it's these children who gather the wood." Most Basotho have balanced expectations of the chores children should perform, which helps protect them from overwork through social surveillance and peer pressure.

When 'M'e Matau was around seven years old, her maternal grandmother asked for assistance, so 'M'e Matau's parents sent her to her grandmother's house. She lived there until she was 15, when her grandmother died. 'M'e Matau viewed her purpose there as work-related but remembered her time with affection. "I was living with her because she was the mother of my mother," she said. "And I think they liked me to stay with her to fetch some water." Although she did perform many household chores for her grandmother, 'M'e Matau was happy to be living there and said that she learned how to be a Mosotho from her grandmother. "Ache," she recalled, "I liked living with my grandmother. . . . When I was living with my grandmother, she was telling me some stories and riddles. And it was nice, and when I went to school, I was telling the other children what I had learned from my grandmother." Other caregivers' recollections of living with grandmothers were almost unanimously positive, producing a kind of collective social memory, a rich tradition already predisposed to see fostering as largely positive and normative. Current fostering practices, shaped by HIV/AIDS, are both a continuation of and a departure from this malleable system of care.

It was not difficult for me to locate families composed of children from various parts of the extended family network. You could knock on any door in rural Mokhotlong and have a fairly good chance of encountering some kind of blended family and an even better chance of finding a household impacted directly by AIDS. However, the importance of ethnographic fieldwork once again became evident in the difficulties I encountered in working to uncover the emotional nature of relationships between children and their nonparental caregivers, since Basotho tended to focus on the physical over the emotional in their caregiving narratives. It was common, for example, for caregivers to talk about the benefits of caring for children by noting their material assistance or economic importance. But through extended observations, I witnessed a strong emotional connection between the majority of caregivers and the children in their care. While love was a major recurring theme in our daily conversations, this discursive love and affection must be understood through a local and culturally mediated lens. A good caregiver was often described as "having love." "I can see that it's his heart," Ntate Kapo's mother said, with respect to his work as a caregiver. Basotho's concept of love is influenced by emotional attachment and shaped by cultural ideas about loving relationships that include the social importance of children, filial responsibility, the social expectation of kin-based care, and the demonstration of love through physical acts of caregiving and reciprocal labor. Affection in this social context is not merely an emotion that exists between two individuals but part of a social norm that has helped protect children orphaned by AIDS.

Grandmothers often cared for their grandchildren, great-grandchildren, or great-nieces and -nephews for reasons born out of necessity and mutual help. Yet the relationship between the young and the elderly goes beyond the practical or the necessary to include strong bonds of affection and love. 'M'e Maliehi, the grandmother of Matseli, claimed that love and experience made old people more fit to care for children. She scolded Ausi Ntsoaki and me, saying, "The young people don't know how to take care of a family. . . . Like you small girls, if you are sent somewhere, you will just take a long time being there. Like going at Janteu [a place for shopping], the sun will set while you are still there not knowing what the children will eat. But me, I will be here always." When I asked her why older people were more willing to provide care for an orphan, she—like many others—claimed, "It's because the old people have love." Later, when we told 'M'e Maliehi that Matseli would be returning to her house after almost a year of rehabilitation at the MCS safe home, she jumped up, did little jig, and sang, "O tla fihla, o tla fihla, abuti oa ka, o tla fihla" (He is arriving, he is arriving, my boy, he is arriving). She spent all day preparing a special meal for him when he returned home.

'M'e Masello and her youngest grandson, Lebo, were also strongly attached. Lebo refused to let anyone else feed him or take him to the bathroom. She told me with frustration, "When he is with the sister at the water tap and when he wants to go *kaka*, he will not tell the sisters. He will just come straight to me and tell me that he wants to go to the bathroom. Sometimes he just soils on himself. And I ask him, 'Why have you done that, yet you were still with your sisters?' He says, 'I didn't want to tell them.' And I become angry. . . . Like even when eating, he wants me to help him, not anyone else. He doesn't want to feed himself." She worried, as grandmothers often do, about what he would do when it was time for him to go to school.

Basotho grandmothers, like many other African grandmothers (Renne 2003), are notorious for spoiling their grandchildren. 'M'e Marefiloe claimed that voluntary fostering had declined because parents did not want their children to be spoiled by their grandmothers. Ntate Kapo, who lived with his two grandsons, described the relationship they had with their great-grandmother, who lived next door. He told me that grandmothers loved their grandchildren as if they were their own children, but sometimes they spoiled them (*ba thefisa*). Thinking of his own mother, he said, "They spoil them; they say, 'Come here, the child of my child.' And sometimes, I have beaten the child because he has done wrong, and the grandmother will be on his side and say, 'Ah ah, I don't want you to do this to my child.' And the children like that about their grandmothers because they know that they fight for them anywhere."

Basotho's (real and idealized) love for children, particularly between grandparents and grandchildren, has been essential in responding to the needs of orphans (Ansell and van Blerk 2004; Young and Ansell 2003). Grandparents increasingly find themselves the only viable caregivers following AIDS-related illness and death. The cultural expectation of affection between grandmothers and grandchildren helps protect and maintain strong intergenerational bonds during difficult times and also helps justify living arrangements outside the patrilineal system. Because of this, a disproportionate number of grandmothers provide care for their orphaned grandchildren—care that requires them to work beyond their physical capabilities, creating loving but vulnerable homes for children.

In addition to the strong intergenerational bonds that exist in Lesotho, an emphasis on good care helps protect orphans from abandonment. Children in Mokhotlong transitioned easily from one household to the next and often found loving and caring environments outside of their natal homes. During interviews, caregivers reported that they would provide orphaned children with care equal to or better than the nonorphaned children living in their households. 'M'e Masekha said that if she could only send one child to school, it would be the orphan because they have no parents.[1] Other caregivers gave a more balanced view of the quality of care, claiming that some caregivers provided good care to orphans, and others did not. 'M'e Masenate, the young caregiver of Tebello (her husband's nephew), was pessimistic that caregivers still living with their own young children could care for orphans with equal attention. 'M'e Maliehi agreed, "The children who are not his or hers will always be working hard," she told me. "Like, if they are two girls—let's say one is hers, and one is not hers—the one who is not hers will always wake up early and do things for the other. And her daughter will do things when she likes." However, when I asked 'M'e Maliehi if there were any people in her village doing this, she said, "*Ache*, no," as if it were more of cultural stereotype of poor caregiving than a common occurrence. Although caregivers may be exaggerating their ability to treat all children as equals, the cultural ideal in caregiving values generosity and empathy over the proximity of the relationship between child and caregiver.

My interlocutors held strong opinions about what makes a "good" caregiver, placing high importance on the physical aspects of care. When caregivers were asked about what a child needs for proper growth and development, they emphasized food, clothing, and cleanliness. "For a child to develop normally," 'M'e Marefiloe told me, "they need to eat well, yes. They need to eat well and to be washed. Like washing her clothes and washing her. And the child will be looking good, if I'm feeding her well and taking good care of her." When children came to town for their appointments at the hospital or when they went to their local clinics, they were always clean and wearing their best clothes. One Friday, while visiting two-year-old Letlo, Ausi Ntsoaki and I counted his pills and found that he was going to run out of antiretroviral medication before his next appointment, which was set for a weekend when the clinic would be closed. We advised 'M'e Mapole, Letlo's grandmother, to set out for the clinic immediately, since the trip would take two hours by foot and taxi and since we were unable to give them a lift, having come via motorcycle. Instead, 'M'e Mapole insisted on bathing Letlo first—even though he looked and smelled perfectly clean— spending the better part of an hour getting water from the tap, making a fire of dried cow dung and brush, and heating water for his bath. She was extremely diligent about keeping Letlo clean, not only for his benefit but as an outward sign that she was a good caregiver.

Although I encountered many examples of excellent care, not all caregivers were able to adequately care for children without support. Poverty and structural inequalities such as poor access to health facilities made it hard for some caregivers to provide for children. Elderly caregivers like Lebo's grandmother struggled due to old age and deteriorating health. The village environment can also be harsh for children with weak immune systems, particularly during the frigid winter months, and children who had been rehabilitated in the safe home, accustomed to a warm sterile environment and a diet high in protein, sometimes became ill shortly after returning to their villages. During my fieldwork, Matseli and Lerato (both HIV positive and both at the safe home for over six months) had to be hospitalized shortly after their return home as they struggled to adjust to the new environment—despite having loving and dedicated caregivers.

High rates of malnutrition, inadequate transportation, and a shortage of material goods (such as household supplies and clothing) also created challenges for caregivers. Sebetsi, age 3 and the youngest of four siblings, lost his mother a year after his birth, and his father did contract work repairing roads for the government, a job that took him away from his four children many days. I visited them three or four times with the outreach workers, and the siblings (the oldest of whom was 10) were always playing by themselves, unbathed, and with torn clothing. In another case, 'M'e Matloane, a young mother and caregiver for her husband's three orphaned nieces and nephews, told me, "Sometimes we go a long time without having any food. And some things like clothes and shoes, and you see that they are not good, and I don't have money to buy new ones, and they delay to have them." Families struggled financially to care for their own children, let alone additional children under their care, and poverty was a common problem. Caregivers frequently worried over lacking money for food, clothes, shoes, Vaseline for dry skin, soap, candles, school fees, and the high costs of funerals. Most caregivers worked hard to care for their children; the challenges they faced were the result not of neglect but of circumstances relating to poverty and a diminished support network.

## CRISIS FOSTERING AND SIBLING SEPARATION

Child fostering in Lesotho is long established, yet the nature of this fostering is currently in flux. For many families now, the movement of children from one household to another is precipitated by a crisis. Crisis fostering is not voluntary but necessitated by emergency situations such as divorce, illness, or death (Page 1989). Networks of care are increasingly strained and saturated, and crisis fostering often occurs in the wake of a mother's hospitalization or death due to AIDS. The special needs required to care for HIV-positive children put physical, emotional, and material strain on caregivers (Heymann et al. 2007; Heymann and Kidman 2009; Singh et al. 2011; Kimemia 2006; Kipp et al. 2006). While crisis fostering can still confer benefits to caregivers and children, the initial motivation for sending children to grandmothers and other kin is no longer companionship or assistance but usually acute need within the family. If there is a healthy grandmother within the family, she is now likely already providing care for other children in need. And yet, families still somehow find a way to make room for more children; over the years, I have encountered very few examples of children being cared for by nonkin or of children being sent to Maseru for institutionalization.

When children are fostered voluntarily in Lesotho, sibling separation often occurs because the circulation of children is enacted as an expansion of social support networks. Many of my interlocutors lived alone with their grandmothers when they were young yet kept close ties with their natal kin and visited often. With AIDS crisis fostering, however, the separation of siblings is more detrimental due to the child's already weakened network of support. Across southern Africa, extended families attempt to keep siblings together, but this is not always possible (Grainger, Webb, and Elliott 2001; Young and Ansell 2003). Among the orphaned children I knew, approximately one-third moved with their siblings, one-third were separated from their siblings, and one-third were only children or had siblings who were grown and no longer in need of care. Among those separated from their siblings, family members decided (often at the funeral of the child's mother or grandmother) that familial resources would be best allocated by separating the children. If they were lucky, like Nkhabu, their siblings would live with another family member in a nearby village. If they were unlucky, their grief at losing their caregiver would be compounded by frequent relocations and sibling separation.

After the death of her mother in 2008, two-year-old Seipati and her two older siblings went to live with their paternal grandmother. Seipati was HIV positive and, due to recurring illness, demanded much of her grandmother's attention and care during the five years she lived with her. At the end of 2012, Seipati's 74-year-old grandmother died, and the siblings had to relocate again. Seipati's two older siblings went to live with their maternal grandmother, but she had suffered a stroke a few years prior and was unable to care for Seipati, whose health had deteriorated. So Seipati was sent along to another village, without the support of her older siblings. Ultimately, Seipati found herself in Maseru, the capital city (a day's travel from her natal village), where she lived with a young maternal aunt who was married but childless. It was likely that Seipati would have to relocate again when her aunt started having children.

Basotho view child fostering not only as a moral good but also as a social responsibility. Familial affection and the expectation that extended kin will care for orphans helps protect children from abandonment or institutionalization. However, AIDS has limited the number of healthy and available caregivers, and children like Seipati often find themselves in loving but unstable homes. The staggering reality of crisis fostering is keenly felt by Basotho, for whom HIV is constantly present. 'M'e Masello saw it when she attended funerals. "There are many more [orphans] now," she told me. "There were not many people dying in the past. But nowadays, week after week, we have a funeral. Week after week, week after week, we just bury many people. Not one person . . . like if it's a woman who dies first, the husband will come after. And if it's the husband who dies first, the wife will come after." Others noted the frequency of grandmothers caring for orphans in their own villages, and most caregivers explained the increase in orphans to AIDS.

Thus far, rural Basotho have not needed institutions to care for children from within their families (and thankfully so—on the handful of occasions in which MCS could not place a child with family, 'M'e Nthabiseng would call the over-crowded orphanages in the city; often she was told that there was no space, or her calls were simply not returned). Despite decades of pervasive pressure on rural communities—and notwithstanding the fact that the grandmothers who have been providing much of the care are aging and dying—families continue to find caregivers for orphans within their own ranks. While fostering relationships no longer follow idealized patrilineal norms, it is still uncommon for people living in Mokhotlong to send their child to live with nonkin.

## CARING FOR AIDS ORPHANS

In addition to the challenges of poverty, structural violence, and crisis fostering, HIV adds a complex layer to the duties of caregivers. While ARVs (antiretroviral drugs) and TB (tuberculosis) medication are free in Lesotho, as are all medications for orphans, transport costs for clinic visits, long distances to health facilities, and other familial responsibilities often put physical and financial strain on caregivers. Caring for a child with acute HIV or associated opportunistic illnesses (such as TB, oral thrush, malnutrition, diarrhea, and severe rashes) is physically and emotionally draining and limits caregivers' ability to maintain employment, complete housework, work in the fields, and care for other children. In addition, the health of the child is often directly related to the health of their caregiver. An undiagnosed and untreated mother often indicates an undiagnosed and untreated child, as children are much more likely to contract HIV from their mother if her viral load is high. I repeatedly witnessed a mother and child deteriorate in tandem. After the death of a mother, then, caregivers are frequently thrust into a situation of initiating treatment and providing care at the height of a child's illness. 'M'e Mapoloko described what it was like to care for Joki shortly after the death of his mother and before he began to receive treatment and financial assistance: "It's difficult to take care of the babies. He was very sick, Joki. He wasn't [healthy] like this. He had a rash. And he had a swollen face like he still has now. He was coughing. He was crying during the day and night. He was scratching himself. And he had diarrhea. . . . Ah, it was difficult, because I was not sleeping during the day and night." Providing 24-hour care would be difficult for anyone, let alone a 77-year-old woman living in a resource-poor setting.

'M'e Masello came to care for Lebo at a particularly precarious time in his illness and had to spend three months at the hospital with him, leaving his brothers and sisters at home. In the children's ward, overworked nurses only provide assistance with doctors' rounds and administer medication and treatments; they do not provide basic care. A caregiver therefore must be present at all times to feed, bathe, and attend to a child. In describing her experience at the hospital with Lebo, 'M'e Masello told me, "He was very sick. He nearly died. He was just like that." She held up three fingers. "And we were admitted at the hospital for this many months." She continued, "I asked for support at the babies house [MCS], not knowing what I'm going to do to feed him because I didn't have anything. He grew up there. He was very sick, *kannete*." Without MCS's help, 'M'e Masello would have not been able to buy food while at the hospital or pay her hospital bills. Her meager pension at that time (200 Maloti per month) was not enough to provide for her household, even before budgeting for Lebo.

Several caregivers also ministered to their daughters during the late stages of their illness, when, lacking care in their husbands' villages, they returned to their natal homes for care, often with a sick child or children in tow. Caregivers recounted these early experiences as particularly challenging. Kotsi, Tsepi, Thapo, Hopolang, and Matseli all returned with their mothers to their natal homes, and all their mothers died shortly afterward. Ntate Kapo described the death of his daughter, Kotsi's mother:

> His mother was married, and she got divorced, and she came back home sick. When she arrived here, I took her to Mokhotlong Hospital. Her stomach was swollen. And when she arrived at the hospital, she was not able to do anything. The nurses told me that my daughter is not taking the drugs, and she refuses to take them. And she said she wants to go to her home. *Kannete*, when I arrived there, I saw her that she wants to fight, she wants to go home, and she wants the nurses to give her the pills to take home. *Kannete*, I agreed, they discharged her, and she came back home. I asked some men to help me to carry her home.... She took three days only, ah ah, there were two, and on the third day, she died. And I passed the message to the parents on the father's side, but they didn't come when I buried her and I cut the *thapo*.[2] And they haven't come even now.

Ntate Kapo had been very close with his daughter, and his mother told me that he cared for her until her death: "She died in his hands. Yes, she died in his hands, the girl." For many families, tension between the maternal and paternal sides is exacerbated by illness and by the affinal kin's perceived failure to properly care for their daughters-in-law in the context of weakened marriages. In several cases, this lack of care was used as justification on the maternal side of the family to assert their right to care for the children.

After their mothers' deaths, each of these children spent time in the MCS safe home for rehabilitation, which is how I came to know them. MCS typically keeps the sickest children for at least half a year, confirming their HIV status, starting them on treatment if necessary, and treating acute malnutrition. Once their health is stable, MCS reunites them with a willing family member, who takes over as the primary caregiver, with visits from MCS every few weeks at first, then monthly. Most MCS clients never live in the safe home, however, so their care and treatment are the caregiver's responsibility from the start. For caregivers of children living with HIV, adhering to a complex medication regimen and attending doctor's visits can be difficult. 'M'e Nthabiseng provided the following insight into the challenges of supporting a child's antiretroviral treatment:

> I think the hardest part is understanding the use of medication and what this medication does to these kids. Because sometimes a kid would have one particular symptom, and maybe through the process where they go see a doctor, whatever, and they end up starting ARVs. So if that one particular symptom—for instance, if there was rash or anything—upon starting medication, if that rash kind of goes away, they kind of feel like, "Oh, that treats rash." So they don't understand that this is the lifetime, these are the doses, do take the meds, we need to come for appointments. Especially with elderly people, illiterate people, it's hard to deal with this medication. Adherence—it's hard. It's really hard. But I think people are trying their best.

Care for a child who is responding well to HIV treatment consists of twice-daily medications of various dosages at the same time every day and a monthly visit to the clinic. But treatment for children is complex because, as children grow, their dosages change. Many caregivers unwittingly make mistakes, and with ARVs, these mistakes can be fatal.

In 2009, one eight-year-old MCS client passed away unexpectedly. Although the immediate cause of the girl's death was not confirmed, her medication had been changed from three separate ARVs to a combination of three medications in a single pill called Triomune. The combined three-in-one pill is designed to help improve adherence, but in this case, the family thought that they were supposed to continue with the old medication as well and for four days doubled her dose. She perhaps did not receive the double dosage for long enough to cause serious harm, but this error illustrates the challenges that loving caregivers face. I was with the outreach team the day we took her body from the mortuary to her village. In the back of the SUV, she lay calm-faced and wrapped in a blanket, which I kept secured to ensure that her body would not roll around in the car. Her family had prepared a rondavel—cleaned and emptied of all furniture—to receive her body, and I could hear the girl's older sister wailing rhythmically in an adjacent rondavel. We paid our respects to the family and left the heartbreaking and unnerving scene, one that repeats too often in Lesotho. The family had spent eight years attending to the girl in loving care, a long time for an HIV-positive child to live, considering that ARVs were not available for the first half of her life. As 'M'e Nthabiseng said many times, people are trying their best, but the complexity of illness and treatment in this environment at times creates insurmountable challenges.

Still, caregivers continue to invest emotionally and physically in infected children. Ntate Kapo described how distraught he was when his grandson Kotsi had to go away to the hospital and MCS: "The most difficult thing is this disease that he has. He had been sick, and I lost hope. I lost hope when he left here." For many years, Kotsi thrived under the excellent care and love of his grandfather. When I would visit his grandfather after their reunification, Kotsi would play nearby, trying to knock the leaves off a tree with a stick or throwing rocks from his garden down onto the road. Every so often, Kotsi would take a break from his game to stand by his grandfather, putting his hand on his grandfather's knee or shoulder to momentarily connect, and then return to whatever energetic game he was playing. Kotsi loved going everywhere with his grandfather, and I frequently spotted the two of them from the road, walking side-by-side in their white gumboots, sticks in hand, trekking up the steep hill to work in their fields. Their relationship clearly brought them both great joy.

Each time I return to Lesotho, I approach the houses of my old friends and interlocutors with trepidation, my heart rate quickening as I knock on the door. My fear is always that the caregiver or child will have died. When I returned in 2013, Kotsi's great-grandmother had died. When I returned again in 2015, I knew something was wrong when I hiked up to Kotsi's house from the road and found long grass growing by the front door. I could see that part of the roof was caved-in as well, notable in light of the loving care that Ntate Kapo had put into his home. I found Kotsi's great-uncle next door. He told me that Ntate Kapo had become sick the previous year and had died after a six-month illness. While my heart sank, I was relieved to hear that Kotsi was living with his mother's brother and a maternal great-uncle in the lowlands. Although I did not see Kotsi in person that trip, his great-uncle told me that the family who took him in had transferred his ART (antiretroviral therapy) to a clinic near his new home, so at least his medical needs were likely being attended to.

The hardships of life in Mokhotlong—often brought on by HIV, exacerbated by poverty—can lead to suboptimal care for children. While it was rare for caregivers to admit to doing a poor job of caring for children themselves, many were able to point to other caregivers who they felt were not managing, based on culturally produced conceptions of acceptable care. Lesotho's Child and Gender Protection Unit (CGPU) is part of the police department (Lesotho Mounted Police Services) and is responsible for dealing with cases of abuse and neglect. Outside of the Maseru district, however, the ability for the CGPU to adequately respond to rural communities is limited by a lack of places of safety, such as MCS's safe home (UNICEF 2009). In most cases, if the police find a neglected or abused child, their only recourse is to threaten the caregiver—there is nowhere to send the child. I only encountered police intervention in child abuse and neglect three times: once when MCS referred a two-year-old boy to CGPU because his grandmother had ceased taking him to ART (antiretroviral therapy) appointments and twice because of abandonment, where the police were attempting to locate the children's mothers to take them to court. In these latter cases, the children stayed at the MCS safe home for a short time, as it is the only temporary residential facility for children in the district. In cases of abuse and neglect, kin-based solutions are not only culturally salient but often the only option.

In the neighboring district of Thaba-Tseka, I met seven-year-old Amohelang, who had severe untreated oral thrush, with open sores all over her lips and tongue.[3] She was on ARVs, and when we counted her medication to ensure that she had enough to get to the next appointment, varying numbers of dirt-covered pills remained in each bottle. Basotho are normally very careful about keeping their homes clean, and health booklets and medication are usually tucked away safely in a plastic bag under a pile of blankets or in a chest. In Amohelang's rondavel, though, flies swarmed on the walls and over large piles of dirty dishes. The floor was littered with empty beer bottles. Her grandmother was there but ignored the unkempt condition of the home. Given these rare outward signs of neglect and considering that even the most loving and well-intentioned caregivers have trouble adhering to the complex ARV treatment schedule, it is doubtful that Amohelang was receiving her medications correctly. It is reasonable to assume that if there were other capable family members aware of her situation, she would not be living with her grandmother.

In 2007, a young boy named Reanetse came to the MCS safe home, extremely ill with undiagnosed HIV. He was treated for almost a year and returned to his home a happy, energetic, and healthy young boy, although his growth was severely stunted. Yet even though MCS paid for his transport to the hospital to receive his medication, his grandmother often failed to come, and when she did, she seemed not to have adhered to his medication regimen. 'M'e Nthabiseng sent the police to talk to her and Reanetse's older sister about taking better care of him, but this produced no change in behavior. Several months later, I checked at the clinic to see if Reanetse had been receiving his medication. He had not.

I knew Reanetse would not live long without his medication—and even if he did resume treatment, having already defaulted several times would severely impact the medication's effectiveness and put him at risk for developing a resistance to the drugs. In this context, 'M'e Nthabiseng made the difficult decision to stop providing services for Reanetse. I pleaded with her to reconsider, but she decided to spend MCS' scarce resources elsewhere, knowing that a supportive caregiver is essential to the health of a child. Without this, further treatment is meaningless. I was never able to determine Reanetse's fate, although I assume the worst. Initially, I struggled with 'M'e Nthabiseng's decision, but I have come to understand the prioritization of services to supportive families. A good caregiver is literally a matter of life and death.

The physical, material, and emotional challenges of care for an HIV-positive adult or child are profound. These challenges are exacerbated by structural issues such as poverty and access to medical treatment and by the complexity of treating HIV in Mokhotlong. Kin-based care is both a culturally salient continuation of a history of fostering and a necessity given the prevalence of HIV in Lesotho. Yet fostering practices have shifted to cope with the changing demographic makeup of the family toward a model that favors and justifies increasing matrilocal care within idealized notions of patrilineality. The emergence of matrilocal care must be understood as firmly embedded in a particular context that is at once open to kin-based fostering but is also structurally constrained by this pervasive health crisis.

## PATRILINEAL DESCENT AND MATRILOCAL CARING PRACTICES

Basotho still hold strong ideals about patrilineal inheritance, marriage practices, and the ownership of children. Despite the flexibility in household makeup in Lesotho, there are rules that guide the decision-making process when determining who will care for children. In theory, if bridewealth has been paid, the father's family has the responsibility—and privilege—of caring for children born to their sons. Children may live with their mother's relatives if both sides of the family agree, but if a child of married parents is orphaned, it is technically the paternal family's responsibility to find the child a home (Murray 1981). Still, as Alber notes in his study of child fostering in Benin, the lived experiences of people are "more flexible and varied than the rules suggest" (2004, 36). Most families in Mokhotlong are surprisingly malleable when it comes to the locality of care and agree that it is best to look at the family situation to ascertain the best environment for a child. Frequently, the mother's family is better equipped (or more willing) to care for a child. More than half the caregivers I worked with were caring for the child or children of a female relative, with matrilocal care negotiated within the patrilineal system. In order to accomplish this, potential caregivers draw on patrilineal rules to make claims for children outside of the patrilineage. As Borneman (1997) and Butler (2002) suggest, people adapt and stretch rules in order to privilege the quality of care over other, more rigid aspects of kinship, such as descent and alliance.

Deciding on a home for a child is often a complex process of negotiation between family members on both sides. If maternal relatives wanted to care for a child, they would invoke often-ignored rules of patrilineality in their negotiations (Block 2014). In numerous cases, young women sick with AIDS returned with their children to their natal homes, and the children stayed on after their mothers died. But the prevalence of maternal caregivers is not merely due to inertia based on the children's location when their mother died; the historical and frequent circulation of children points to Basotho's ease with this movement. Instead, weakened marital relationships and the importance of affectionate care have led to this recurring pattern.

In many examples presented here, failure to pay bridewealth was the cultural lynchpin on which maternal caregivers based their claims, even though it is common in the current economy to marry without it. Couples sometimes married without even intending to pay bridewealth, yet the strength of the cultural practice and the generation of older adults for whom it remains important mean that the ideal is ever-present and potentially in play for any marriage. 'M'e Matau, for example, wanted to keep her grandchildren in her care, so she argued that they belonged to her since the husband's family "never sent cows." She claimed that the paternal grandparents did not really want the children and that their claims of affection were merely empty talk. She believed their motivation was purely economic: "They just want to eat with them. They just want these children to work for them." By claiming the in-laws merely wanted to "eat with" (e ja ka) the children, she negatively linked the children's labor to their livelihood. Although there was obvious affection between 'M'e Matau and her grandchildren, she also recognized the value in their labor, telling me, "I like them to help me because I have been caring for them." Yet 'M'e Matau presented the paternal grandparents as unethical, claiming their request for the children was not also accompanied by genuine love and care, which further helped strengthen her social (as opposed to legal) claims to the children.

Ntate Kapo's effort to secure caregiving responsibility for three-year-old Kotsi and his brother also relied on a claim about bridewealth; again, the lack of care by the paternal kin was this maternal grandfather's primary concern. Like many young women, Kotsi's mother returned home during her illness and passed away under her father's care. One time, I asked Ntate Kapo about following kinship rules in general and, unprovoked, he used the opportunity to explain why it was his right to care for Kotsi and his brother:

And now let's say their mother came with them, and she was very sick, do you hear? Let me tell you. Her marriage was already not good. She was not living well when she was coming here. And I was the one looking after her until I took her to the doctors and she died. And after she died, I called her parents-in-law [*babohali*], but they did not come. And I did all the things by myself [for the funeral]. And they came after some months, saying they are coming to take the children, and I asked them, "The children of whom? Because you did not even pay *likhomo*." Because they did not even come when the mother died. And they went back without anything. They didn't have anything to do. They would not take me to the court because they did not pay *likhomo*.

I was curious about Ntate Kapo's emphasis on following the rules of "Sesotho culture," given his living arrangements as a maternal caregiver—and a man at that. On several occasions, he emphasized that orphaned children should go to their father's side, so I inquired about situations where matrilocal care was justified. "In Sesotho culture," he told me, "they should be in agreement with the parents to show that their children have gotten married. And if there is no marriage, it is as if she was just living with him only. And she will come back at her home." Trying to draw him out, Ausi Ntsoaki asked how one would know that the couple was married: "If *likhomo* are there," he explained, "if that person has paid *likhomo* to show that he is married." He told us that the only way a child could go to the mother's side is if bridewealth had not been paid, positioning himself as a strong enforcer of rules since it allowed him to show how the paternal family did not follow them perfectly—something he was well aware was rare.

'M'e Malefu's case had certain similarities to Ntate Kapo's, as she was caring for her daughter's two school-aged girls. Her daughter had been married with the expectation that the "cows would follow," however, the family was unable to pay, so 'M'e Malefu claimed that they were not married. She too made the claim that the in-laws were not caring for her daughter and had failed to attend her funeral. Unlike Ntate Kapo, however, she and her husband went to court to legalize their claim for the children, even though the paternal relatives sent a letter from their chief saying that 'M'e Malefu could have the orphaned girls. Ausi Ntsoaki and I were curious about why she took this legal precaution in the face of the paternal family's apparent lack of interest in the children, so I asked if her daughter was married.

'M'E MALEFU: *Ache*, yes, but she was stolen, then after they were not able to pay *likhomo*, so she was not married. . . . And when she was sick, they were not taking care of her until she came back home. And after that, I was the one caring for her. And they didn't come at all. I took her to the hospital until she died. Even when she died, they didn't come for the funeral. The children were at the house where she was married. And we went there and asked for them because their father died before the mother. And we went to the court, and we told those people that we want our children because the parents of their father did not pay *likhomo*. And they gave us the children. And we came with them here.

ELLEN: Did the paternal grandmother also want to take the children?

'M'E MALEFU: No, they didn't say anything. They were told when my daughter died, but they didn't come. My husband called them to the court and showed that he wanted the children because the parents on the father's side didn't like his daughter. And they didn't pay *likhomo*, and he didn't think they would take good care of her children.... Even the letter that was given by the chief [from the father's side] said the grandparents don't have a problem if we take the children.

ELLEN: Why did you have to go to court if the other family didn't even want them in the first place?

'M'E MALEFU: We went to the court because we wanted things to be certified. Not to agree only. We wanted something which certified that we have taken the children.

'M'e Malefu repeatedly mentioned that bridewealth had not been paid—this was her legal claim to the children. Yet she emphasized the lack of care by the paternal family as her primary motivation for legal actions. Despite the formal separation of Sesotho laws and government laws in Lesotho, 'M'e Malefu used both customary and formal legal structures to achieve her particular social ends. In this case, the legal claim reinforced the kinship claim, which was fundamentally about quality of care.

There is the potential, however, that the legal and kinship claims might contradict each other, as seen in the story of Matseli and the Ntho family, which opens the book. Like many other families, Matseli's mother migrated with her children to her natal home during the late stages of her illness, when both she and Matseli were quite sick with AIDS. Ntate Kanelo, Matseli's grandfather, levelled a familiar accusation about the care his daughter received while ill. "The parents on the father's side were not taking care of the mother," he said. "They were not taking care at all." Yet Ntate Kanelo and 'M'e Maliehi felt deeply insecure about the lack of formality in their arrangement to care for the grandchildren. "When we die, what is going to happen?" he asked. "Because we don't have a boy. What is going to happen to our houses? I don't know." While Ntate Kanelo was concerned that they had no boy to inherit their property, 'M'e Maliehi was worried about the children's care, each of them focusing on their gendered areas of responsibility. "Me, I just think what if *Ntate-moholo* and I, we can both die, who is going to take care of these children of my daughter?" she said. "Because we are the ones taking care of them. Because, on the father's side, they seem not to take care of them.

And I'm always praying to God to help me so that I can live for a long time and they should be old enough to do things for themselves." I told 'M'e Maliehi that I hoped she would live a long time too, and she laughed wistfully.

Although the paternal family had shown no prior interest in caring for the children, the Ntho family harbored concerns that they would try to claim them in the future. "Because we are the parents of their mother, we have to take care of them," Ntate Kanelo said. "When they grow up and if they want to go to that family [father's side], they will go because they are still using their surname." The unspoken concern was that once the children were old enough to contribute significantly to the household, especially in terms of agricultural work, the paternal family would want them back. The paternal family's insistence on burying Matseli at their home—which they did in a paltry grave with no funeral—was the family's attempt to signal ongoing attachment to the children and to cling to the threads of patrilineal duty and decency, if only slightly. The Ntho family's substantial caregiving investment and deep emotional attachment was not enough to ensure that the children belonged to them, since at the time of marriage, the husband's family paid four cows, an acceptable initial payment. While the remainder of the agreed-upon bridewealth was never paid, this partial payment created significant insecurity for the Ntho family.

The emphasis on bridewealth payments in negotiating caregiver rights is notable because bridewealth is increasingly uncommon among Basotho. Historically, it reinforced the processual nature of a union, where an initial payment was made at the time of marriage, and the remaining cows (or agreed equivalent of cash, goods, or other animals) were paid over time (Murray 1981; Ashton 1967). Contemporary marriages, though less reliant on bridewealth, are nonetheless conceived of as a process, not a single event (Comaroff and Comaroff 2001; Townsend 1997), and while many Basotho participate in legal and customary marriage ceremonies, others consider cohabitation to signify the start of their marriage. Thus the marital status of a couple, and therefore the appropriate caregiver for orphans, is open to negotiation.

Elderly Basotho are more likely than young people to extol the virtues of bridewealth in strengthening a marriage and, conversely, to attribute the dissolution of marriages to the decline in bridewealth practices. Several elderly Basotho told me that when they fought with their spouses, their parents encouraged them to "have patience" (ba le mamello). Here, she reinforced the popular view that bridewealth creates bonds between affinal kin that make divorce more difficult. Young people living in rural areas or those who self-identified as traditional were more likely to share these views about bridewealth. For example, 42-year-old Ntate Kalasi, who had promised six cows but only provided two (which he paid in cash) before his in-laws died, said that marriages would be stronger if bridewealth was paid. He believed that "men would be crying for their cows," therefore, working hard to stay in their marriages in order to keep the bridewealth in the family. Unlike the elderly people who lamented the decline in bridewealth and the decrease in its monetary worth, 'M'e Mapole, a young mother, was realistic about current economic constraints while still seeing value in the symbolic exchange: "Paying *likhomo* [cows] doesn't mean the kraal should be full of them. But if you have paid one, it's enough. Even if it wasn't the same as in the past, but it should be paid. Because most of the people can't pay that amount that was paid in the past. There are few people who can pay that now." Turkon (2003) notes that current bridewealth practices utilize a variety of strategies in negotiating the tradition. Where bridewealth payments of any size were previously the norm, they are increasingly the exception. Furthermore, not all caregiving arrangements are negotiated based on the presence or absence of bridewealth. Two of the grandmothers I knew cared for their daughters' children even though bridewealth had been paid, at least in part. In contrast, I knew several paternal grandmothers who were caring for their grandchildren even though bridewealth had not been paid.

In the current context of marital instability and illness, many young people are choosing to have children outside of marriage. In 2009, 51.5 percent of men and 34.3 percent of women (ages 15 to 49) in Lesotho had never married. Yet the fertility rate remains high, especially among rural populations, at an average of four births per woman (Lesotho Ministry of Health 2016). When I first began to work in Lesotho, I asked for paternal information as part of standard household data collection. If a girl was unmarried, the common survey response was that the father of her child was "unknown." These nominally "fatherless" children are disadvantaged in that the disassociation with their paternal kin reduces their potential networks of kin-based support. However, this also allows young women to participate in childbearing, which is still important for most women (Booth 2004; Pearce 1995), while protecting the natal kin's status as the primary caregiver during uncertain times.

The animosity that can develop between families during child-care negotiations can create problems for children. Reamohetse was forced to go from caregiver to caregiver as her family argued about who was best suited to care for her. Meanwhile, her father and aunt, who lived adjacent to each other, were fighting because the father had taken Reamohetse back to his home without discussing it with the aunt, then wanted the aunt to take her back when he realized that he was doing a poor job of caring for her. Ultimately, Reamohetse's father would have liked her to live with a sister in South Africa who was already caring for another one of his daughters, but he was trying to get the appropriate papers when he was put in prison, and this wish never came to pass. When I last saw Reamohetse, she looked thin and unhappy and cried whenever she was not being held by her aunt.

Caregivers must navigate various pressure points when deciding on the locality of care for children. The intricate dynamics of negotiations are complicated by the expectation that children will be a potential source of labor as they age. The caregivers' anxieties examined here stem at least in part from the potential for lost labor, although in many cases, the child's long-term survival at the time of household migration was not assured. In other words, the future is often too uncertain to plan around. Additionally, while the care of young children costs a great deal of time and energy and demands intensive caregiving, the care of older children requires considerable financial investments in education. Families engage in contested negotiations about who will care for orphans since children are highly valued by Basotho, but caregivers are in short supply. The current trends in caregiving arise from the ways that people regard their social and moral obligations to kin, their desires to care for children, and the extremely limited resources most families in Mokhotlong have to devote to another dependent child.

## CONCLUSION: THE SHIFTING LANDSCAPE

Basotho children move easily between kin for various social and economic reasons, with an emphasis on nurturing strong bonds between grandparents and grandchildren in order to facilitate mutual assistance. However, the form and function of fostering in Lesotho has taken on new dimensions as HIV/AIDS limits family members' ability to care for children and increases the responsibility of caregivers for the needs of HIV-infected and -exposed children. Furthermore, pervasive poverty and structural inequalities make the additional costs of orphan care challenging for many families.

As I have illustrated, HIV/AIDS has substantially undermined Basotho families' capability for kin-based foster care. More children are in need of care, yet fewer caregivers can provide it. In rural communities where institutionalized care is virtually nonexistent and government and NGO support is limited, kin-based care remains the only option. To cope with these pressures, families are organizing themselves by focusing on matrilocal resources, even while making sense of this model of care within the context of an idealized patrilineal system of fostering. Families therefore attempt to demonstrate their right to children by focusing on the presence or absence of bridewealth, depending on which position they wish to take. At the same time, there is an overriding emphasis on the quality of care that potential caregivers can provide.

The day-to-day role of women—particularly elderly women—in this system has not drastically changed. Women still do most of the carework, despite a growing number of male caregivers (for more on this, see Block 2016). Women are being called upon to care for an increased number of children—including those with greater health problems—with fewer resources. What has changed, however, is the role a woman's natal family plays in supporting her. Families are pooling their resources with their daughters instead of their sons. In conformity with the conceptualization of "official kin," the rules of child fostering are rigid and fixed, but in practice, child fostering is flexible and allows for a wide range of household configurations. Caregivers who are trying to legitimize their right to care for a child emphasize its rigidity because it allows them to point to the ways in which other potential caregivers are subverting these rules. Matrilocal caregivers must negotiate for the care of children while maintaining the dominant patrilineal ideology of care. Caregivers thus have been able to represent "practical kin" as if they were "official kin," legitimizing matrilocal care within the patrilineal system. In this way, women are simultaneously reinforcing the patriarchal structure of the Basotho family and resisting it to accomplish one of their most important social roles: caregiver.

# CONCLUSION
## Infected Kin

## Hopolang the Runner[1]

*When I was walking home from school today, I saw a lizard scurry across the rocks—one of those tiny cute ones, the greeny-orange ones you can see when it rains. Nkhono hates those lizards too much, swatting with her broom and yelling Haie mona! Whenever she found one in our rondavel, she would make me chase it away. If it was raining, she wouldn't come inside until first I made sure it was gone. Hele!—she was afraid, grandmother, but not me. It's silly how adults can be scared of tiny things.*

*I am not afraid of anything. Not lizards, ghosts, witches, or even thokolosi. When I was smaller, my sisters tried to make me cry with stories about thokolosi, but I am 11 now. I am the fastest girl in standard five, faster than everyone but three boys, and I am too big to be fooled by those stories for babies.*

\* \* \*

*At lunchtime today, some of the other girls were singing "Miss Lucy Died." In addition to being the fastest runner, this is something else I'm famous for: I taught that song to my whole school. Now everyone knows it. It was a song I learned from my lekhooa when she used to visit from America, back when I was maybe five years old. Palesa would have been 10, and Mosa 12, and they would help me take my medicine. But when my lekhooa started visiting us in my village, she showed us that they were not giving the medicine properly. She was telling nkhono and my sisters all kinds of things about that disease and about how to use Sekhooa medicine. That is something makhooa love: always running around talking Chivee! Chivee! Chivee!*

*One time, she came to the rondavel when I was playing with my friends, doing that Sakurumba dance, and she wanted to know what it meant. We tried to explain, but how can you even say what the words to a song mean? I told her the part*

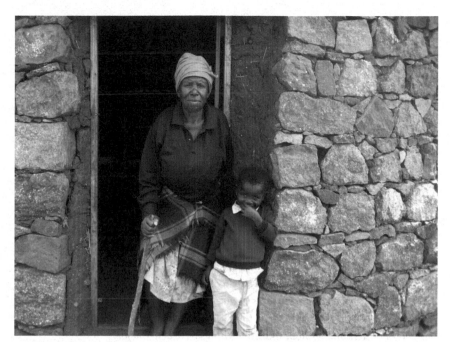

FIGURE 5.1. Hopolang and her great-grandmother, 'M'e Mamorena, Mokhotlong, 2008

*O jele moroko! O jele litsila!*, *and my friends were laughing at me. You just do the dance—that's it.*

*After we showed her* Sakurumba, *she showed us the dance from America called "Miss Lucy Died," and we fell* down, *we were laughing so hard. It is one thing to have a* lekhooa *coming to talk to you in your house, but that dancing—ah ah!—it was too much. My* lekhooa *was very funny, and she was always happy even though she had no children. She would bring me little presents, some sweets and soaps and candles for the rondavel. When we would hear her coming on her motorcycle,* nkhono *would say, She is coming on her horse! Every time, she said it, that same joke.* Nkhono *is very kind and funny, but she only knows one joke.*

\* \* \*

*I was just a small girl when my mother died.* Nkhono *says we came to the village when my mother was sick from that disease, but I don't remember any of it. Palesa and Mosa probably remember something, but they never tell me. I can't remember my father either, but once I heard* nkhono *talking about him—she said he went off to work in Natal before I was born, and no one has heard from him since. But that was a long time ago.*

*When my mother was sick,* nkhono *was taking care of her day and night, and then after she was gone, my sisters and I stayed there in the village with* nkhono. *This was the kind of thing my* lekhooa *was always asking about—lots of things about Sesotho culture, like why do kids go to this side and not that side, why, why, why? Nkhono told her that when the mother is gone, the children must stay on the father's side. That way, if the mother wakes up in her grave, she will come looking for us at that place. If the children are in the wrong place, the mother will just be asking, "Where are my children? Have you lost them?"*

*My mother never came looking for us, at least I don't think so. But how could you even recognize the ghost of someone you don't know?*

* * *

*Last night, I woke up when it was still deep, deep night. The dogs were barking like crazy outside, like they were really scared of something. I rolled over to get closer to* nkhono, *and then I remembered she was gone.*

*From the corner of my eye, I could see something moving in the dark by the wall, but I didn't want to look. I pressed my face against the mat, then sat up quickly and looked where the thing was moving. There was nothing.*

*After a moment, I closed my eyes again. The only other sound was 'M'e Bohobe snoring across the room. She is kind to me, but this house in Mapholaneng is empty without my sisters and without* nkhono. *Things were better before.*

* * *

*One time, my* lekhooa *came to visit us when we were taking maize kernels off the cob, so we decided to make* liqhome *for her. She loved that popcorn too much, maybe because they don't have it in America. But when she told* nkhono *what she wanted to talk about that day, my grandmother told us to go outside. We pretended to go, but instead we listened under the window, because when someone says to go outside, you can be sure you need to hear that thing.*

*Palesa and Mosa were laughing so hard, but quietly, so we wouldn't be discovered. I was laughing too, but truthfully I didn't understand what they were talking about. Then my sisters told me what a man does with his thing and how you can put that plastic on it. In Sesotho, you can call that plastic* khohlopo, *which means gumboot, and that is what my* lekhooa *was talking about in there. Nkhono kept saying, "I want to see it. . . . I haven't seen it, and I want to see it!" and Palesa and Mosa were laughing harder and harder, because how can those things even be for old people?*

*But really* nkhono *was very good at knowing about that disease and helping me. When I was still small, the village health worker was telling other people about my status, and all the children and adults knew about it; everyone was whispering and gossiping. Then* nkhono *confronted the village health worker, yelling,* Why are you saying this thing and that thing about Hopolang! Nkhono *said she would fight that woman. Really, everyone knew it was just talk because* nkhono *was already very weak, but that woman stopped whispering things about me.*

My sisters were helpful too, telling me when to take my medicine, but even they could forget sometimes. Soon I was doing everything myself. I knew all the times to take the medicine and the right amounts too. When I was nine, I was going to the clinic myself, not even with my sisters. I was just running alone.

I remember one time when I forgot to take those pills before school, and nkhono was so angry—but the truth is that I didn't forget. I had to race my friend to school that day, and I already said I am the fastest girl. I wasn't going to lose that race. When I got home, nkhono was sitting in the shade under the peach tree where she always waited for us. Hei!—she was so angry, knocking her cane on the ground and saying, Hopolang, I will beat you! so I had to run inside and hide from her, calling out, I forgot, nkhono!

But I was very careful after that. Even if I was playing somewhere else, I would come home to take those pills. I knew them all perfectly.

\* \* \*

This is how I became the fastest runner.

When we would go to church with nkhono, she was always walking so slowly. Even then her knees were painful—ichu!—she was suffering! I would run to the church and then run back, and nkhono was in the same place. Then I would run again to the church and back, and still she had barely moved. On Sunday, I was just running and running all day.

Nkhono said I was a blur.

\* \* \*

Tonight, I woke up and was lying in the dark, hearing those dogs barking, when I realized it happened again. I had to sneak around the room, trying to wash off the mat, the whole time thinking 'M'e Bohobe was going to wake up and ask me, Hopolang, what are you doing?—but how could I even explain that those baby things were happening in the night? Like I should be wearing nappies!

I think if 'M'e Bohobe really woke up, I would just run from the house.

It was too embarrassing.

\* \* \*

But I can say this about 'M'e Bohobe: she always makes sure I have sugar in my porridge, even if it is not as good as when nkhono made it.

\* \* \*

Not like Uncle.

Kannete!—I hate that man.

\* \* \*

When my grandmother was getting too sick, we had to send for 'M'e Bohobe to help us. Palesa and Mosa and I were caring for nkhono, cooking papa and lijelello and gathering wood, fetching water from the tap and washing dishes, doing laundry—all those normal things—but soon it was too much. Nkhono was really suffering, coughing so much and having chest pains. But even when she was dying, we were still sleeping in the room with her. Kannete—we wanted to stay with her! Then 'M'e Bohobe came to help us, and soon after that, nkhono was called home.

All the family came to the funeral so they could decide where my sisters and I should go. Uncle said we had to come with him. He was shouting at 'M'e Bohobe, saying, "Who do you expect will cook for me when you have all these children?" So we had to go with that drunk man. We were staying with him for three months—ache!—he was treating us very badly there. Then one aunt came from Qwaqwa and took Palesa with her. She knew Uncle was killing us the way we were living. She didn't want us to stay there, but she couldn't take all three of us.

After Palesa was gone, I told Mosa it was our turn to leave. Uncle was going to starve us, using all that money for alcohol. But Mosa was loyal or afraid or what? She was 18. I don't know what she was planning; she only said she would stay there.

I told her I wouldn't let that drunkard kill me. I told her I was the fastest runner, and so I ran all the way to 'M'e Bohobe's house. Never once did I look over my shoulder.

* * *

For some months, 'M'e Bohobe and I were waiting for Mosa to join us. First, she told 'M'e Bohobe that she was staying with Uncle so she could finish standard seven, and then she would leave so she could go to high school. But when the holidays came, she never appeared.

We didn't know where she was. Later we heard that she had gone far off to Qwaqwa and had been married to an old man there. Someone told us she was the sixth wife. Three previous wives had died, but two others were still living, and now Mosa was a wife as well.

I will never get married. No one will be fast enough to catch me. Sometimes, at night, when nkhono was singing to us and telling us old riddles and stories, she would say that we should never marry. Go have babies if you want, she said, but when you get married, you are only living badly with these men who do nothing.

I don't know why Mosa went to Qwaqwa. Maybe she thought that was the only way to escape Uncle, or maybe she just had to. But she should have stayed with me.

* * *

In my whole life, I only fought with nkhono one time, when I was still a small girl. We were cooking in the rondavel, and nkhono asked me to bring some porridge over to her, but when I picked it up—ichu!—that porridge burned me so badly! Right away,

*I knew she had tricked me for not paying attention. I ran out of the rondavel crying and holding my hand, then went to the tap to run water over it.*

*I was so angry at nkhono. All day I wouldn't talk to her, and even at night, she was singing me extra songs, and still I refused to speak. I didn't want to forgive her. That is the only time I can remember being upset at her, truly.*

*But I'm careful now. Nkhono did teach me that lesson. I know some pots will burn you when you don't take care.*

\* \* \*

*You can understand things differently when you are big. Now I know nkhono was trying to prepare me for this time when she would be gone, even though I didn't understand it when I was small.*

*Once, I can remember, I was watching nkhono make the morning fire, and she was really suffering, crying out from pain when she was moving around. I was maybe six. I told her, "Nkhono, if you die, I can go to the camptown and live there. And when you come back, I will come back." She was just looking at me when I said this. After a while, she said, "Ah ah—when I'm dead, I won't come back. You won't see me again, my child, you will just remember me." I told nkhono she was wrong, that God would make her survive, but still she was just looking at me. Then she asked me to go fetch water.*

*And we do remember her. Whenever I see those tiny lizards, I think about her. And I always remember how she was kind to me and how she told me stories at night. When it is harvest time, 'M'e Bohobe and I set aside food for her so nkhono can know she is being treated well. And sometimes she visits me in my dreams.*

-WM-

\* \* \*

## AIDS IS A KINSHIP DISEASE

HIV/AIDS is undeniably a biomedical illness, yet its impact goes far beyond an individual patient's physical response. AIDS scholars have long noted the impact that kinship and culture have had on the epidemic in southern Africa, yet most studies on the ways in which culture and sociality influence HIV/AIDS only examine the illness through the narrow lens of a particular intervention's success or failure. With this approach, HIV/AIDS is assumed to be the stable component of the equation, bolstered by its biomedical assertiveness, and culture is seen as the external (and often irrational) influence that maps onto the biomedical facts and hampers intervention. The prevailing logic, in other words, is that the problem could be solved if only culture didn't get in the way. Furthermore, the deeply embedded structural inequalities that lead to global health inequalities are so comprehensive and so time-consuming to repair that they are taken as inevitable, leading to narrow vertical interventions pursued even when they are understood to be insufficient. Yet the research I have presented in this book shows that the intersection of HIV and kinship must be understood as a mutually reinforcing dialectic, encompassing factors like caregiving practices, social relationships, cultural ideas about illness, and political, economic, and historical circumstances. The context of rural Lesotho directed the course of this illness though its population and transformed the disease itself. AIDS is a kinship disease because kinship and AIDS influence each other at the most profound and hidden levels of sociality.

Several important recent works have addressed a trend toward what has been called "AIDS exceptionalism," where AIDS becomes the health issue of concern even when its prevalence is low—a result of the privileged position AIDS has occupied in global health and development circles, where funding priorities are set. Adia Benton (2015), in her penetrating book, shows how HIV predominates in the imaginaries of development experts and ordinary Sierra Leoneans, even as its prevalence remains at less than 2 percent of the nation's population. Daniel Jordan Smith notes that—although the HIV prevalence rate in Nigeria hovers around 3 percent—there too AIDS looms in the social imagination as a "symptom and a product of a collective moral crisis" (2014, 2).

In Lesotho, as elsewhere, AIDS has become a proxy for other social moral concerns—in particular the changing social order and the failures of kinship more broadly. Yet what is exceptional about AIDS in Lesotho, unlike in many West African countries, is that the HIV prevalence rate remains astonishingly high, at around 23 to 25 percent, where it has stagnated for more than a decade (Lesotho Ministry of Health 2016). In Lesotho, the effects of HIV/AIDS are felt in each household and in every rural corner of the mountain kingdom. The illness is an integral part of everyday life, leaving no family unscarred. While Nigeria has many more people living with HIV, due to its significantly larger population, HIV does not pervade the landscape in the same totalizing way that it does in Lesotho. More insidious than the high rates of illness, however, are the ways in which HIV intersects with kin-making methods that are fundamental to cementing social relationships, spreading through sexual intercourse and the life-giving processes of birthing and feeding.

Despite the quantitative and qualitative differences of AIDS in Lesotho as compared to countries with lower prevalence rates, Lesotho has not been immune to the drawbacks of AIDS exceptionalism. Nora Kenworthy's ethnography of HIV initiatives in Lesotho demonstrates how efforts to scale up HIV interventions and services have failed patients in innumerable ways, including by depoliticizing them and by creating what she calls a "politics of recipiency" (2017). Kenworthy shows how the single-minded focus on AIDS has moved attention away from other important social ailments and from the broader failures of the health system. As Weigel and his colleagues (2013) argue, health initiatives that narrowly target a single disease in the Global South are problematic: they do nothing to strengthen health infrastructure, they fail to address the underlying structural inequalities that allow future health problems to flourish, and they neglect the ongoing persistent health problems such as malnutrition and food insecurity that have threatened marginalized populations for decades. Instead, scholars have argued for a diagonal approach to global health, with initiatives aimed at strengthening the infrastructure of health systems even as they work toward improving outcomes for specific health targets (Weigel et al. 2013; Shiffman 2009).

The problems of scope and scale that plague global health interventions also create imbalances in global health research. Work that focuses narrowly on the physical ailments of patients and takes place only in clinics and hospitals—where biomedical concerns are emphasized—ignores the social context in which the majority of daily experiences take place. It is essential, then, to focus on the lived realities of individuals as members of families and communities. It is likewise necessary to look beyond everyday practices to the contemporary and historical global economic and political forces that impact human health and "threaten the social fabric" of communities (Goodman and Leatherman 1998, 5). As I have demonstrated, the AIDS epidemic does not merely threaten this social fabric but fundamentally restitches it.

In recognizing the larger forces at play, I have kept unequal structures at the forefront of the analysis by incorporating a broader historicized view of Lesotho's emergence and growth as an enclave nation and a remittance economy. Yet the microlevel lens that predominates in this book draws into sharp focus how structural inequalities affect individuals and communities. Everyday negotiations and practices around illness, kinship, and care intersect with broader structural factors such as access to treatment and migrant labor. A narrow focus on either microlevel individual practices or broader sociopolitical structures would miss the important connections between these realms of investigation.

Idealized notions about kinship (including lineality and locality of care) are often presented as inflexible in Lesotho. In practice, though, these notions are far more adaptable to social change. Rural Basotho have used this flexibility to accommodate the pressures that emerged with the onset and proliferation of HIV/AIDS. The most readily identifiable example of this involves an increasing emphasis on the centrality of the house as a stable fixture in Basotho social and economic life. In its simplest form, the house is a place where people live and where fundamental acts of kin-making—birthing, caring, feeding, and raising— take place. But the house is more than merely a space where these acts of sociality unfold; rather, it is where people "dwell." The "dynamic" and "processual" nature of the house is key to producing and reproducing social relationships

(Carsten and Hugh-Jones 1995). In this way, the house mimics the dialectic relationship between HIV and kinship. Neither HIV nor the house is a discrete entity that maps onto Basotho people's everyday experiences and understandings of kinship; both are actors in the production of those experiences and meanings. The house is a focal point of this book because it reflects the social and political-economic context in which people live. Adults and children move between households because of employment, illness, and caregiving; during this time of transition, the social geography of the house provides a good milieu in which to analyze these movements. These microshifts in the configurations of people who share the space where kin ties are shaped help illuminate the macrochanges in social organization.

In exploring these movements, I noticed a marked shift toward matrilocal caregiving practices. Despite continued patrilineal ideals, in practice, orphans are increasingly cared for by maternal relatives. The tensions between ideal and practice are highlighted in the negotiations that take place when caregivers make claims to care for orphaned children. Paradoxically, matrilocal caregivers often position themselves as strong believers and enforcers of idealized rules of patrilineality. By doing so, they are able to legitimize their roles as caregivers by demonstrating how the paternal family has failed to adhere to the same rules. One specific area where this frequently occurs is with the fading institution of bridewealth. Even though bridewealth payments are in decline, maternal caregivers argued for their caregiving rights by pointing to the ways in which the paternal family has fallen short in this idealized transaction. The growing orphan population, combined with a shortage of healthy caregivers, has changed the way care takes place in Lesotho. Rather than following a prescribed set of rules, families seek to find the best possible caregiver in terms of willingness, health, emotional attachment, and economic means. This flexibility has resulted in an increase in maternal caregivers—particularly maternal grandmothers—for AIDS orphans. Although strong notions about lineality and kinship can be limiting, they can also be leveraged to create legitimacy for a variety of caregiving and household arrangements.

On their own, any of these adjustments by families would be interesting but perhaps not warrant claims about a fundamental shift in the way Basotho kinship works. However, when observing this changing landscape as a whole—from the practical arrangements of care to the changing ideas about lineality—the fundamental and profound ways that AIDS has become a kinship disease are clear. This raises a pressing question: since all major illnesses change the ways in which families live, what makes something a kinship disease? I contend that a kinship disease alters processes of relatedness not just for a few families but for a population of people, reverberating beyond the person who is sick and impacting all members of the community. AIDS has altered social and familial life in Lesotho, and Basotho kinship can no longer be explained without it.

## BEYOND LESOTHO AND AIDS

The focus of this work has been the everyday experiences of Basotho women and men in context. The vivid accounts of the successes and challenges of AIDS orphans and their families give color and context to the intersection of HIV and kinship in this particular place and time. I depict a range of Basotho people's experiences and emotions and gain depth and texture from literary non-fiction vignettes—our attempt at an "anthropology of the whole." By necessity and by choice, this work is deeply contextual; however, the findings I present reach beyond the mountains of Mokhotlong—and even Lesotho—to provide insight into other areas of theory, research, and practice. If qualitative research is to be more than merely anecdotal, it must have some transferability—results generalizable to other contexts and settings (Lincoln and Guba 1985). Although the data are intended to give the reader an intimate understanding of the local, the theoretical and empirical findings presented here have both localized and broader transferability.

Studies from other areas of southern Africa note many of the same broad concerns regarding the social implications of HIV, the impact of migrant labor on communities, and the importance of kinship and sociality in responding to AIDS interventions. In particular, those interested in rural southern African communities with high HIV rates and large orphan populations will benefit from the theoretical and empirical findings of this research. This is important: 19 million people—more than half of global HIV infections—live with HIV in southern and eastern Africa (UNAIDS 2017). HIV impacts kinship practices, household dynamics, caregiving relationships, treatment-seeking behaviors, and encounters with health care providers. Work that acknowledges this deeper embeddedness at all levels will lead to a genuine understanding of people's beliefs and behaviors surrounding HIV. The intimate and microlevel view of everyday practices in family life that ethnographically ties this book to highland Lesotho can be replicated in multiple contexts.

In a regional context, I have illuminated the potential areas where ideal-ized notions about kinship and care might mask coping strategies in everyday practice. As I suggest, we need to explore this delicate balance between cultural flexibility and cultural constraint. Strict idealized notions about gender, lineal-ity, and caregiving should be interrogated to reveal diverse coping strategies. Comparative studies between southern Africa and other global contexts could be productive regarding the intersection of HIV and kinship. These comparative inquiries may shed light on locally specific HIV/AIDS epidemics and could build on the theory of AIDS as a kinship disease in unexpected ways. Further, the idea of a "kinship disease" could apply to other locales and illnesses; comparisons between HIV and other widespread health problems might lead to interesting and profound insights about human experiences of debility and disease. Beyond illness, the negotiations that take place between real and idealized notions of kinship and gender in particular would be useful to examine in any number of contexts, especially those that highlight individual- and community-level strengths in dealing with adversity, poverty, structural inequalities, and marginalization.

Practice theory is useful in thinking through how everyday actions and negotiations lead to systemic change. Sherry Ortner, a strong proponent of practice theory, has expanded on the work of Pierre Bourdieu in order to illuminate how everyday actions lead to cultural change. She argues that while practice is thought to increase individual agency, real social change is, for the most part, "an unintended consequence of action" (1984, 157). In this case, I illuminate the matrix where culture, illness, and care intersect to explain how individual- and community-level strategies during a protracted health crisis have led to a shift toward increasingly flexible notions of lineality. Changes in Basotho kinship strategies occur not because people decide a cultural overhaul is needed but because the minute negotiations and subtle but pervasive shifts in how people care for children within the family eventually add up to a changed system through changed practices. It is the gradual shift, out of population pressure and necessity, which leads to social change. In Mokhotlong, this manifests in the centrality of care as an organizing principle of social life, the primacy of the house in shaping relatedness, and the emerging practice of families pooling resources around their daughters' children. Elsewhere, the examination of everyday practices and negotiations could illuminate the ways that major social disruption can lead to broader social change, including people's responses to conflict, forced migration, or natural disasters.

It is clear that social relationships play a significant role in determining health outcomes in marginalized communities. Lesotho's AIDS-orphan crisis and the challenges that caregivers face offer insight into Basotho coping mechanisms and show how the pandemic has impacted families and communities. I originally undertook this project with vague notions about the ways that sociality and kinship interact with health and care, yet as my investigation advanced, the deep intersections of HIV and kinship became ever more visible. It is my hope that this work helps others understand these profound connections and approach research and interventions—in southern Africa and beyond—with renewed insight into the benefits of a fully biocultural approach to global health inequalities.

## POSTSCRIPT: ANTICIPATING THE CHALLENGES
## OF GRANDMATERNAL DEATH

We began this chapter with Hopolang's story because it highlights many of the important findings of this book: the deep intersections of AIDS and kinship, the intimate relationships between grandmothers and grandchildren, the flexibility of kinship and gender, and the profoundly human and diverse ways that people cope with crisis. Yet we also began this chapter with Hopolang's story because of the way it ends—with the death of her grandmother. I began investigating the impact of grandmaternal death in earnest during my last two trips to Lesotho, in 2013 and 2015. But my interest in this potential shift began in 2010 when, a few months after returning home from a year of fieldwork, I got a call from 'M'e Nthabiseng. She paused in the middle of our phone conversation and then told me abruptly, "Lebo's grandmother has died." In the conversation up to this point, I had thought she sounded less effusive than her usual bubbly self, but I chalked it up to the poor signal that often made phone calls to Lesotho challenging. Afterward, I realized that she had been working up to this news. She knew that I had a particularly close relationship with 'M'e Masello and Lebo, the child whose HIV diagnosis shifted a number of times over the years (see the vignette at the beginning of chapter 3).

'M'e Masello was an exemplary caregiver. She was affectionate, diligent, and self-sacrificing toward Lebo and his siblings. She was also an anthropologist's dream—welcoming, chatty, hyperbolic, and indignant. She was a natural storyteller who loved to hold court, telling tales of how much food and *joala* they had served at a family funeral, exploring the intimate details of Lebo's miraculous "cure" and reversal, gossiping about the time that cousin of a neighbor stole books from the school. But she suffered from chronic asthma and other undiagnosed chronic ailments—perhaps chronic obstructive pulmonary disease (COPD)—for many years and was frequently in and out of the hospital, leaving Lebo's teenage sister to look after him and the other siblings. So while it was no surprise that she had died, I wondered who would care for Lebo now. The negotiation for his care several years prior at his mother's funeral had been difficult, and I worried that the paternal family might reject him. Fortunately, they willingly took in Lebo and his siblings and transferred his antiretroviral treatment to the clinic nearest their village—a good indication that they would attend to his health.

'M'e Masello's death triggered a host of other big questions: If grandmothers were caring for the majority of orphans, who would care for them as grandmothers started to die in greater numbers, as they certainly would? Would the kin-based networks of care that had been deemed saturated finally collapse, as many had long suspected? Would an increasing number of children be sent to the few, overcrowded orphanages in the city? Would siblings be separated? Or would families continue to adapt in order to provide care within their homes? And if families did take these children in, what kind of care would they receive and from whom? I returned to Lesotho to find out what happens when grand-mothers die.

When I began this new line of inquiry in 2013, I encountered a methodo-logical problem. I was looking for interlocutors who were no longer living. I reasoned that if I could find any children not living with their mother or a grand-mother (great-grandmothers included), it was likely that there was no available grandmother to care for them. I was correct. In 2013, I located 20 nongrand-maternal caregivers fostering a child.[2] In all but two cases, their grandmothers were not available because of death, ill health, or an already overwhelming caregiving burden. In 2015, I surveyed 200 households living with orphans and found a similar pattern. Of the 378 single and double orphans in this survey, the majority were living with either their mother or their grandmother. Still, orphaned children were more likely to live with another relative (such as an aunt or older sibling) than nonorphaned children (32 percent as compared to 13 percent). Additionally, only one-third of children who had lost their mothers and who had a living grandmother were not living with them. This rate dropped to one-quarter when considering only available maternal grandmothers. So grandmothers—especially maternal grandmothers—overwhelmingly remain the first-line of defense in the absence of a mother.

On my most recent trip to Lesotho, in 2015, I encountered another meth-odological problem I had not anticipated—this time an emotional one. In the year-and-a-half interval between fieldwork trips, a number of the caregivers who I had known for many years had died. Some deaths were expected, such as the nonagenarian great-grandmother in chronic pain who told me at my last visit, "I want to die. I want God to take me so I will not be suffering anymore." Others, including Kotsi's young grandfather, Ntate Kapo—who was in his 60s and who I had known since 2007—passed away unexpectedly, leaving behind two orphaned grandsons. Ntate Kapo was very dear to me, and I approached his boarded-up house with my stomach in knots, a dawning realization that my research life and personal life were, at times, indistinguishable.

Hopolang's story exemplifies the challenges of grandmaternal death in rural Lesotho. Kinship networks struggle to withstand demographic pressures on the family, and changes do not occur seamlessly. When I visited 'M'e Mamorena in 2013, she looked a decade older than when we had met three years prior. I asked her if she had a plan for the time when she could no longer care for Hopolang and her sisters, delicately broaching the subject of her impending death. She didn't flinch: "When I die, the family will take care of the children. They will sit down and say, 'Here are the children.' So they will ask that boy [referring to her adult grandson], 'Is there anyone who will take responsibility when *nkhono* has died?'" When I asked whether her grandson showed an interest in taking the children, she lamented, "No, he doesn't care about them. He doesn't take any responsibility . . . this boy doesn't ever visit, and his wife never visits either." I wondered if she was worried that the girls would not be well cared for. "It hurts my heart," she said starkly. "I am worried. But there is nothing I can do."

'M'e Mamorena died a few months later, although I did not find out about her death until February 2015. When I approached her house on a beautiful sunny day and found her usual spot under the peach tree empty, my excitement at our reunion drained away. Her family told me that while her joints continued to bother her, her chest pains from the edema worsened until she died at home after a painful two weeks in September 2013. As with many families, the conversation about who would care for the children occurred at the funeral, which, as her daughter-in-law proudly informed me, was widely attended by family and neighbors. As 'M'e Mamorena suspected, the children's care fell to their father's brother and his wife, who were living in a nearby town. However, as the opening vignette in this chapter shows, the uncle was a drunk, unable to provide adequate care, and the children fled in various directions.

Hopolang and her sisters' experience highlights what can happen when grandmothers—who have cared for orphans in the time of highest AIDS mortality—age and die. In addition to the loss of their primary and beloved caregiver, Hopolang and her sisters experienced increased migration, sibling separation, and decreased quality of care. While their uncle seemed to have his own personal problems to contend with, an increasing number of men in Lesotho are woefully underprepared for the care work they find themselves performing (Block 2016). Of course, many men do excellent work. As one grandfather (rather tellingly) explained, he cared for his grandsons "like a mother." Others, like Hopolang's uncle, buckle under the weight of their responsibilities or exploit young girls for household labor or both.

In Lesotho, the resilience of kinship networks and the availability of grandmothers are two primary reasons kin-based care for orphans did not collapse during the first decade of the 21st century, when AIDS mortality was at its peak. However, as the current cohort of elderly caregivers dies, the potential for social dissolution looms—this time without the safety net of grandmothers. In other words, grandmaternal care may have merely postponed a caregiving crisis. While this population shift is in its infancy, kin-based care networks continue to dominate caregiving. In the absence of grandmothers and other older female relatives, however, Basotho are reconfiguring their relations again to care for their children. This reorganization comes at a cost: families look to younger women and inexperienced men to care for children. And as Hopolang's experience shows, orphans are experiencing increased separation from their siblings and multiple migrations between households within the extended family. These shifts will impact orphans and their caregivers' health, age at marriage, educational attainment, and other markers of well-being and development. Now—over two decades into the AIDS epidemic in Africa—it is clear that AIDS's impact goes well beyond the sick individual, pervading the entire social network. While researchers and funding bodies are experiencing AIDS fatigue, the ongoing and ever-changing nature of HIV demands our continued attention. Grandmother mortality is merely one of these challenges.

# ACKNOWLEDGMENTS

I have left the task of writing the acknowledgments until the last possible moment, because I was waiting for the inspiration to write something beautiful and moving that would convey my deep gratitude and affection for the people who helped make this book possible. I am now realizing that it will never be possible for me to do justice to those with whom I worked—my interlocutors, my mentors, my supporters, and my coauthor—so the thanks that follow will have to suffice.

First, I need to thank the many Basotho grandparents, parents, caregivers, and children whose stories fill the pages of this book and whose names cannot appear here. The heart of this book is grounded in their words and experiences, and it is their joys and struggles that fill the book with hopefulness and life. I am entirely indebted to the staff at MCS (Mokhotlong Children's Services) for putting up with my incessant questioning and for providing me with insights and friendship over the past decade. In particular, thanks to 'M'e Nthabiseng, my lifelong friend and supporter, whose bird dance and *lilietsane* always beckon me back to Mokhotlong. And to her son, Tumo, who is like a big brother to my own children (who frequently pester me about when *abuti* Tumo is coming to visit again). I am grateful to my friends who visited me in the field: Tasha, Liz, Jenn, and Steph. And to Nastassia Donoho, who tracked down an excellent photo-op for me. I also give special thanks to my research assistants, especially Ausi Ntsoaki, for her constant companionship and insight and for trusting me with her life day after day by climbing onto the back of my motorcycle. Finally, thanks to the MCS fellows with whom we lived, especially Reid and Bridget, who endured the world's longest double date with us and who became our lifelong friends.

My most sincere gratitude also goes out to my dissertation committee at the University of Michigan. I somehow had the great good fortune of assembling a team of brilliant, kind, and supportive women from both anthropology and social work: Elisha Renne, Karen Staller, Gillian Feeley-Harnik, Holly Peters-Golden, and Letha Chadiha. Your insights and improvements are all over this book, and you all somehow made your criticisms sound like encouragement. Your influence on my work is indelible and enduring. I am also thankful for the enriching intellectual environment at Michigan and the many other graduate students and faculty who helped make me into an anthropologist, in particular Kelly Fayard, Elana Buch, Laura Heinemann, and Jess Robbins, who all share my love of kinship; my social work cohort, especially my dear friend Becky Karb;

and Mandy Terc, my writing partner, generous reader, and friend. Any graduate student of my era at Michigan would also be remiss if they did not give thanks to the inimitable Laurie Marx, cheerleader to all.

At Brown University, where I did a two-year postdoctoral fellowship at the Population Studies and Training Center (PSTC), I am grateful for the companionship of my colleagues, especially my cubicle-mates Kelley Smith, Jo Fisher, and Andy Fenelon; my writing group, including Adia Benton, Melissa Hackman, and Jennifer Stampe; and my idea-bouncer extraordinaire, Trina Vithayathil. I am also grateful for the rich intellectual environment of both PSTC and the anthropology department, as well as the outstanding mentorship of many, especially Sherine Hamdy, who encouraged me in pursuing a rich ethnographic approach; Bianca Dahl, whose insightful comments led to new areas of inquiry; Dan Smith, who opened many doors (and wrote many letters); and Jessa Leinaweaver, my kinship guru, most helpful reader, and friend.

I was very fortunate to land at the College of St. Benedict and St. John's University with a wonderful group of colleagues and supporters, especially Sheila Nelson, Jeff Kamakahi, Jessy O'Reilly, Megan Sheehan, Michael Rosenbaum, and Sheila Hellermann (who makes all our lives infinitely easier). And of course, I have much gratitude for my students, whose openness to new ideas and passion for social justice give me hope for the future.

My work in Lesotho was made possible by financial support from a number of places. I am grateful to the W. K. Kellogg Family Endowed Fellowship, whose generous support funded the bulk of my dissertation research. I am also grateful to the Department of Anthropology and the Rackham Graduate School at the University of Michigan for their financial and bureaucratic support over the years. This work was also generously supported by the Fulbright U.S. Scholar Program and by the Population Studies and Training Center at Brown University. The PSTC receives core support from the Eunice Kennedy Shriver National Institute of Child Health and Human Development (5R24HD041020).

I am so pleased to be publishing this book in the fabulous series at Rutgers titled Medical Anthropology: Health, Inequality, and Social Justice. Thanks to the anonymous reviewers, whom I cannot thank in person but who will see their imprint on this book in many important ways. Kimberly Guinta has been an outstanding and accommodating editorial director. I am also eternally grateful to Lenore Manderson. Within 30 minutes of meeting Lenore in 2013, she had already roped me into numerous fascinating projects. She personifies what it means to be a mentor: she works constantly to amplify her mentees, many of whom are women, and she measures her value as a scholar by how much she is doing for her younger colleagues. I look forward to seeing what she cooks up for me next!

Finally, I would like to thank my family: my many parents, Sheila, Howard, Julia, Jim, and Joannie; my siblings, Emily and Dan; and my children, Sam, Eve, and Mara, who bring so much joy to my life (and to all the people—family and otherwise—who have cared for them while I worked on this book). And to my partner-in-crime, coauthor, editor, and inventor of truly innovative dance moves, Will, who has made this book come alive with his magic.

~Ellen Block

\* \* \*

I am grateful first to the Mohlomi family and to Lineo Shata, both of whom were generous with their time and patient with my questions.

Thanks are also due to Lineo Segoete and Nthabeleng Lephoto, who brought keen eyes to my words and gave crucial editorial guidance.

Much gratitude and love go to my colleagues at Seeiso Griffiths in Mokhotlong, who taught me—well, pretty much everything.

Many thanks to Lenore Manderson and Kim Guinta, who through tireless application of intellect and heart willed this book into existence.

And to Ellen, of course—who brought me there, who makes each day better than the last.

~Will McGrath

# GLOSSARY OF SESOTHO TERMS

**ache:** an exclamation indicating frustration

**abuti:** brother

**ausi:** sister

**Basotho:** the people of Lesotho (sing. Mosotho)

**bukana:** health booklet

**chobeliso:** the practice of stealing a woman from her village to marry her, abduction

**Famo:** Sesotho music, usually with vocals, accordion, drum, and bass

**genitor:** from Latin, indicating a person's biological father

**hae:** an exclamation, similar to "Hey!"

**hele:** an exclamation, usually celebratory

**joala:** home-brewed Sesotho beer

**Kwaito:** South African house music

**kannete:** an exclamation or verbal pause, used for emphasis, similar to "I swear!"

**khohlopo:** gumboots or rubber boots, slang term for condoms

**lekhooa:** a white person or foreigner (pl. makhooa)

**lerato:** love

**lesheleshele:** porridge

**likhomo:** cows, bridewealth

**'M'e:** mother, or Mrs.

**makoenya:** fat cake

**makoerekoere:** derogatory racialized term used to describe foreign black Africans

**mamello:** patience

**mohlaba:** Sesotho beer, when brewed for the purpose of honoring ancestors

**mokaola:** a local illness category characterized by a wide variety of symptoms, thought to be HIV in the early years of the epidemic

**moroho:** Sesotho dish of seasoned chopped greens, eaten with maize meal

**Mosotho:** a person from Lesotho (pl. Basotho)

**ngaka ea Sekhooa:** biomedical doctor, usually meaning white or foreign doctor, lit. "English" doctor

**ngaka ea Sesotho:** Sesotho doctor, indigenous healer

**ngoaneso/ngoanaka:** my sibling, also used as a term of endearment akin to "my dear"

**Ntate:** father, or Mr.

**Ntate-moholo:** grandfather, lit. old father

**Ntate Molimo:** God the Father

**Nkhono:** grandmother

**papa:** maize meal, Lesotho's staple food

**pater:** from Latin, indicating a person's social father

**phatsa:** to make incisions on the body where medicines are rubbed, used by indigenous healers

**pitso:** community meeting, usually organized by the village chief

**rondavel:** a Sesotho round house made of stones, a thatched roof, and floors and walls plastered with a mud-and-dung mortar

**Sesotho:** language of Lesotho, culture of Lesotho

**Sotho-sotho-sotho:** an expression meaning very Sesotho or traditional

**thapo:** a strip of black cloth that mourners wear around their necks

**uena:** you

# NOTES

## INTRODUCTION

1. This vignette previously appeared in a somewhat different form in *Everything Lost Is Found Again*, © Will McGrath, included with permission from Dzanc Books. An earlier version also appeared in *Asymptote*, April 2013.

2. ARV (antiretroviral) drugs refer to the three-drug cocktail that make up ART (antiretroviral therapy).

3. *Mosotho* is singular for a person from Lesotho (plural is *Basotho*).

4. Life expectancy, which had slowly risen from 46 in 1960 to 59 in 1990, reached a low of 44 in 2003 (Lesotho Ministry of Health 2010). Since the spread of ARVs, it rose to 48 in 2013 (UNDP 2013).

5. In 2014, only 59 percent of men and 38 percent of women were employed (Lesotho Ministry of Health 2016).

6. Much has been written about HIV/AIDS in South Africa and the AIDS denialism that characterized the first decade of the AIDS pandemic there. For excellent discussions of these issues, see Fassin (2007); van der Vilet, Kaufmann, and Lindauer (2004).

7. Free ARVs and associated medications are available at all public health facilities, including hospitals and clinics. However, if a patient chooses to go to a private clinic, they will pay for the doctor's consultation.

8. For example, 38 percent of all public and private health facilities in 2006 were located in Maseru, which houses only 23 percent of the population (Mwase et al. 2010).

9. An AIDS orphan is defined as a child who has lost one or both parents to AIDS. While some AIDS orphans are infected with HIV, most of them are not.

10. Customary laws in Lesotho, also known as the Laws of Lerotholi, were compiled in 1903 and focus both directly (through laws about rights and duties of heirs) and indirectly (through laws on inheritance related to the chieftainship, land use, and property) on children (Juma 2011).

11. A rondavel is a small, round house found throughout Lesotho and in South Africa. Our rondavel was built by local contractors with cinderblocks and cement instead of rocks and mud and had a thatched roof made of wheat stalks. See chapter 1 for more about Basotho houses.

12. Sesotho is a Bantu language that is spoken primarily in Lesotho and by a small proportion of South Africans. It is virtually impossible to learn Sesotho in American institutions, so while I studied as many texts and guides as possible before conducting fieldwork, most of my language acquisition occurred while in Lesotho with the help of tutors, research assistants, friends, and interlocutors. While I can speak conversational Sesotho and have a sizeable vocabulary, I am nowhere near native fluency, so I conducted interviews with a research assistant. Ausi Ntsoaki acted as my primary translator until 2009, and 'M'e Mamosa and Ausi Lieketso took over the job in 2013 and 2015. My interlocutors were most comfortable in their native tongue, so the majority of these interviews were conducted in Sesotho, although I often conducted interviews in English with MCS staff, social workers, and health care providers. My research assistants and I transcribed interviews together, painstakingly going through

each recording, discussing the possible meanings of certain words and expressions, and checking each other's work.

**13.** *Makhooa* is plural, and *lekhooa* is singular. In Sesotho, pluralization occurs at the beginning of a word.

**14.** In Lesotho, *makoerekoere* is a derogatory racialized term used to describe foreign black Africans, though usually not those from South Africa, Botswana, or Swaziland. The origins of the term are unclear, but some claim it is an onomatopoeic word mimicking the sound of unfamiliar African languages (Obioha et al. 2012; Akokpari 2005).

## CHAPTER 1     KINSHIP FIRST

**1.** See amendments to the Land Act of 1979 (Larsson 1996) and the Legal Capacity of Married Persons Act of 2006 (Mapetla 2009).

**2.** Lesotho has the lowest fertility rate in southern Africa. Rates have decreased from 5.4 births per woman in 1976 to 3.3 births per woman in 2014 (3.9 in rural areas, 2.3 in urban areas; Lesotho Ministry of Health 2016).

**3.** *Ache* is a common Sesotho exhortation used to add dismay or regret.

**4.** The use of teknonyms is optional. Once a woman changes her name after the birth of her first child, she will use this name throughout her life. Guma (2001) states that men also take teknonyms in Sesotho culture, but I never witnessed nor heard of this practice.

**5.** Shortly after arriving in Lesotho, foreigners are offered names by their friends or acquaintances. My Sesotho name, 'M'e Makeletso, was given to me by 'M'e Nthabiseng, the managing director of MCS.

**6.** Many of these naming practices exist in other African cultures. For example, Zulu names often express the circumstances surrounding a child's birth or the emotions the parent is feeling at the birth of the child (Suzman 1994).

**7.** Because the elderly are highly respected in Sesotho culture, their funerals are widely attended.

**8.** *Joala* is brewed by women and is used for everyday social and ritual purposes. It is also a primary source of income for women not otherwise employed. See also Spiegel 1981; McAllister 1993; Saul 1981; and Karp 1980.

**9.** Only elderly Basotho eat the food plated specially for the ancestors.

**10.** Customary law dictates that upon divorce, a woman's family is required to return the *likhomo*, and she must return to her natal home with only her personal possessions. If there are children, they must remain with their father's family (Gill 1994). In practice, this is much more flexible.

**11.** Heidegger, in "Building, Dwelling, Thinking" (1971), explores the relationship of building to dwelling. He emphasizes the role of dwelling to our situated place in the world and to our very "being." While earlier studies of houses expanded our understanding of a "building" perspective, these insights are not rendered insignificant by a "dwelling" perspective. Rather, the two approaches are synergistic.

## CHAPTER 2     MEDICAL PLURALISM IN A LOW-RESOURCE SETTING

**1.** CHAL is part of the larger U.S.-based NGO Global Ministries, which is run by the Christian Church (Disciples of Christ) and the United Church of Christ. CHAL is funded by numerous local and global donors and also receives money from the Lesotho government.

2. My experiences were consistent with a country report from Médecins Sans Frontières (2007).

3. Christian-run organizations in Africa have been widely criticized for their approach to mitigating HIV, specifically with respect to abstinence-only education, discouraging condom use, and AIDS denialism (Campbell, Skovdal, and Gibbs 2011; Prince 2009; Parsitau 2009). Here, however, I am merely focusing on the comfort that religion provided to many caregivers with whom I worked.

4. While malaria is not endemic to Lesotho, malaria treatments would be among the frequently treated illnesses elsewhere in southern Africa, where HIV/AIDS and TB rates are also high.

5. This type of exchange is partly driven by a cultural deference and respect for authority figures and partly because Lesotho is not a society that values question asking. This was particularly evident when observing child rearing. Basotho children learn by observation and are often chastised when asking too many questions. My occupational predilection for asking questions was tolerated with forbearance, though not always appreciated.

## CHAPTER 3    "LIKE ANY OTHER DISEASE"

1. Voluntary counseling and testing counselors are government-trained employees who do pre- and posttest counseling as well as perform and record the results of HIV tests. They are employed at every hospital and clinic, including mobile clinics.

2. Data on HIV prevalence among the elderly is limited. UNAIDS (Joint United Nations Programme on HIV/AIDS), one of the primary sources of global AIDS statistics, only provides age-specific data for people under 50. According to data from 2004, Basotho men in their 50s had an HIV-prevalence rate of approximately 16 percent. However, in a South African study from 2008, the HIV-prevalence rate for men and women over 60 was 3.5 percent and 1.9 percent, respectively, suggesting that the rate drops precipitously after the age of 60. However, the current generation of HIV-positive adults is aging and living longer because of ARVs, so research with this population group is needed (Negin and Cumming 2010).

3. Trimethoprim-sulfamethoxazole is the prophylactic (such as cotrimaxazole, or Bactrim) taken daily by ART patients in order to prevent opportunistic infections.

4. Gumboots are tall rubber boots worn by many Basotho, particularly shepherds. The use of khohlopo to refer to condoms is likely borrowed from the British term rubbers, which refers to both boots and condoms.

5. Serodiscordance is when one member of a couple is HIV positive and the other is HIV negative.

6. Until 2010, the Lesotho government did not start pregnant women on the full course of ART but started them on AZT (azidothymidine) in their 28th week of pregnancy.

## CHAPTER 4    ORPHAN CARE AND THE FAMILY

1. In reality, 77 percent of double orphans in Mokhotlong attended school, while 91 percent of children living with at least one parent attended school (Lesotho Ministry of Health 2016).

2. Thapo is a strip of black cloth that mourners wear around their necks. It is cut approximately one month after the funeral.

3. Oral thrush is an opportunistic infection associated with HIV that results in sores around and inside the mouth. It is a clinical sign of advanced HIV that physicians often use to initiate treatment if a CD4 (cluster of differentiation 4) count is unavailable.

## CONCLUSION

1. Almost all details in this story come from interviews, field notes, and direct observation; anything in quotation marks comes directly from transcripts. Other statements have been paraphrased slightly for the sake of narrative felicity. Most details from Hopolang's internal monologue are taken from comments she made to Ellen or to her grandmother and are documented in the transcripts. However, in a few instances, I made imaginative leaps concerning the exact nature of Hopolang's thought processes—but not without the consultation of several female Basotho readers as to their accuracy and authenticity. The majority of this book privileges the voices and perspectives of caregivers. My intention in telling this story from Hopolang's point of view at the end of the book is to give voice to those most affected by the continuing challenges of AIDS orphaning, including the deaths of grandmothers.

2. Of this group of 20 caregivers, 13 were young women in their childbearing prime, mostly aunts and sisters from both sides of the family, and 7 were men (5 grandfathers, 1 uncle, and 1 brother).

# REFERENCES

Adato, Michelle, Suneetha Kadiyala, Terence Roopnaraine, Patricia Biermayr-Jenzano, and Amy Norman. 2005. "Children in the Shadow of AIDS: Studies of Vulnerable Children and Orphans in Three Provinces in South Africa." International Food Policy Research Institute, Washington, D.C.

Adichie, Chimamanda. 2009. "The Danger of a Single Story." TED video, 18:43. Filmed July 2009. http://www.ted.com/talks/chimamanda_adichie_the_danger_of_a_single _story?language=en.

Akokpari, John K. 2005. "Strangers in a Strange Land: Citizenship and the Immigration Debate in Lesotho." Development Southern Africa 22, no. 1: 87–102.

Alber, Erdmute. 2004. "Grandparents as Foster-Parents: Transformations in Foster Relations between Grandparents and Grandchildren in Northern Benin." Africa 74:28–46.

Alverson, Hoyt. 1978. Mind in the Heart of Darkness: Value and Self-Identity among the Tswana of Southern Africa. New Haven, Conn.: Yale University Press.

Ansell, Nicola, and Lorraine van Blerk. 2004. "Children's Migration as a Household/Family Strategy: Coping with AIDS in Lesotho and Malawi." Journal of Southern African Studies 30, no. 3: 673–690.

Ashton, Edmund H. 1967. The Basuto: A Social Study of Traditional and Modern Lesotho. London: Oxford University Press.

Babb, Dale A., Lindiwe Pemba, Pule Seatlanyane, Salome Charalambous, Gavin J. Churchyard, and Alison D. Grant. 2007. "Use of Traditional Medicine by HIV-Infected Individuals in South Africa in the Era of Antiretroviral Therapy." Psychology, Health and Medicine 12, no. 3: 314–320.

Baer, Hans A., Merrill Singer, and John H. Johnsen. 1986. "Toward a Critical Medical Anthropology." Social Science and Medicine 23, no. 2: 95–98.

Bahloul, Joëlle. 1996. The Architecture of Memory: A Jewish-Muslim Household in Colonial Algeria, 1937–1962. Cambridge: Cambridge University Press.

Beidelman, Thomas O. 1972. "The Kaguru House." Anthropos 67:690–707.

Benton, Adia. 2015. HIV Exceptionalism: Development through Disease in Sierra Leone. Minneapolis: University of Minnesota Press.

Bhengu, Busisiwe R., Busisiwe P. Ncama, Patricia A. McInerney, Dean J. Wantland, Patrice K. Nicholas, Inge B. Corless, Chris A. McGibbon, Sheila M. Davis, Thomas P. Nicholas, and Ana Viamonte Ros. 2011. "Symptoms Experienced by HIV-Infected Individuals on Antiretroviral Therapy in Kwazulu-Natal, South Africa." Applied Nursing Research 24, no. 1: 1–9.

Biehl, Joao. 2005. Vita: Life in a Zone of Social Abandonment. Berkeley: University of California Press.

Bikaako-Kajura, Winnie, Emmanuel Luyirika, David W. Purcell, Julia Downing, Frank Kaharuza, Jonathan Mermin, Samuel Malamba, and Rebecca Bunnell. 2006. "Disclosure of HIV Status and Adherence to Daily Drug Regimens among HIV-Infected Children in Uganda." AIDS and Behavior 10:S85–S93.

Birdwell-Pheasant, Donna, and Denise Lawrence-Zúñiga. 1999. "Introduction: Houses and Families in Europe." In *House Life: Space, Place and Family in Europe*, edited by Donna Birdwell-Pheasant and Denise Lawrence-Zúñiga, 1–35. New York: Bloomsbury.

Bledsoe, Caroline. 1989. "Strategies of Child-Fostering among Mende Grannies in Sierra Leone." In *Reproduction and Social Organization in Sub-Saharan Africa*, edited by Ron J. Lesthaeghe, 442–474. Berkeley: University of California Press.

———. 1990. "'No Success without Struggle': Social Mobility and Hardship for Foster Children in Sierra Leone." *Man* 25, no. 1: 70–88.

Block, Ellen. 2014. "Flexible Kinship: Caring for AIDS Orphans in Rural Lesotho." *Journal of the Royal Anthropological Institute* 20, no. 4: 711–727.

———. 2016. "Reconsidering the Orphan Problem: The Emergence of Male Caregivers in Lesotho." *AIDS Care* 28, no. S4: 30–40.

Bohannan, Laura. 1952. "A Genealogical Charter." *Africa* 22, no. 4: 301–315.

Booth, Karen. 2004. *Local Women, Global Science: Fighting AIDS in Kenya*. Bloomington: Indiana University Press.

Borneman, John. 1997. "Caring and Being Cared For: Displacing Marriage, Kinship, Gender and Sexuality." *International Social Science Journal* 49:573–84.

Bourdieu, Pierre. 1977. *Outline of a Theory of Practice: Cambridge Studies in Social Anthropology*. Cambridge: Cambridge University Press.

Boyer, Pascal, and James V. Wertsch. 2009. *Memory in Mind and Culture*. Cambridge: Cambridge University Press.

Bray, Rachel. 2003. "Who Does the Housework? An Examination of South African Children's Working Roles." *Social Dynamics* 29, no. 2: 95–131.

Bulled, Nicola. 2014. *Prescribing HIV Prevention: Bringing Culture into Global Health Communication*. New York: Routledge.

Butler, Judith. 2002. "Is Kinship Always Already Heterosexual?" *Differences* 13, no. 1: 14.

Campbell, Catherine, C. A. Foulis, S. Maimane, and Z. Sibiya. 2005. "The Impact of Social Environments on the Effectiveness of Youth HIV Prevention: A South African Case Study." *AIDS Care* 17, no. 4: 471–478.

Campbell, Catherine, Morten Skovdal, and Andy Gibbs. 2011. "Creating Social Spaces to Tackle AIDS-Related Stigma: Reviewing the Role of Church Groups in Sub-Saharan Africa." *AIDS and Behavior* 15, no. 6: 1204.

Carroll, Vern. 1970. *Adoption in Eastern Oceania*. Honolulu: University of Hawaii Press.

Carsten, Janet. 1991. "Children in Between: Fostering and the Process of Kinship on Pulau Langkawi, Malaysia." *Man* 26, no. 3: 425–443.

———. 1995. "The Substance of Kinship and the Heat of the Hearth: Feeding, Personhood, and Relatedness among Malays in Pulau Langkawi." *American Ethnologist* 22:223–241.

———. 2004. *After Kinship: New Departures in Anthropology*. Cambridge: Cambridge University Press.

Carsten, Janet, and Stephen Hugh-Jones, eds. 1995. Introduction to *About the House: Levi-Strauss and Beyond*, 1–46. Cambridge: Cambridge University Press.

Carsten, Janet, ed. 2000. Introduction to *Cultures of Relatedness: New Approaches to the Study of Kinship*, 1–36. Cambridge: Cambridge University Press.

Cheney, Kristen E. 2017. *Crying for Our Elders: African Orphanhood in the Age of HIV and AIDS*. Chicago: University of Chicago Press.

Chigwedere, Pride, George R. Seage Iii, Sofia Gruskin, Tun-Hou Lee, and Max Essex. 2008. "Estimating the Lost Benefits of Antiretroviral Drug Use in South Africa." *Journal of Acquired Immune Deficiency Syndromes* 49, no. 4: 410–415.

Chimwaza, Angela F., and Susan C. Watkins. 2004. "Giving Care to People with Symptoms of AIDS in Rural Sub-Saharan Africa." *AIDS Care* 16, no. 7: 795–807.

Chitereka, Christopher. 2009. "The Challenges of Social Work Training: The Case of Lesotho." *International Social Work* 52, no. 6: 823–830.

CIA. 2017. "World Fact Book: Life Expectancy at Birth." Accessed May 24, 2018. https://www.cia.gov/library/publications/the-world-factbook/rankorder/2102rank.html.

Clark, Shelley. 2004. "Early Marriage and HIV Risks in Sub-Saharan Africa." *Studies in Family Planning* 35, no. 3: 149–160.

Cocks, Michelle, and Anthony Dold. 2000. "The Role of 'African Chemists' in the Health Care System of the Eastern Cape Province of South Africa." *Social Science and Medicine* 51, no. 10: 1505–1515.

Cohen, Rachel, Sharonann Lynch, Helen Bygrave, Evi Eggers, Natalie Vlahakis, Katherine Hilderbrand, Louise Knight, Prinitha Pillay, Peter Saranchuk, and Eric Goemaere. 2009. "Antiretroviral Treatment Outcomes from a Nurse-Driven, Community-Supported HIV/AIDS Treatment Programme in Rural Lesotho: Observational Cohort Assessment at Two Years." *Journal of the International AIDS Society* 12, no. 2: 23–30.

Comaroff, Jean. 1985. *Body of Power, Spirit of Resistance: The Culture and History of a South African People.* Chicago: University of Chicago Press.

Comaroff, John L. 1978. "Rules and Rulers: Political Processes in a Tswana Chiefdom." *Man* 13, no. 1: 1–20.

Comaroff, John L., and Jean Comaroff. 2001. "On Personhood: An Anthropological Perspective from Africa." *Social Identities* 7, no. 2: 267–283.

Cooper, Elizabeth. 2012. "Sitting and Standing: How Families Are Fixing Trust in Uncertain Times." *Africa* 82, no. 3: 437–456.

Coplan, David B. 1987. "Eloquent Knowledge: Lesotho Migrants' Songs and the Anthropology of Experience." *American Ethnologist* 14, no. 3: 413–433.

———. 2001. "A River Runs through It: The Meaning of the Lesotho–Free State Border." *African Affairs* 100, no. 398: 81–116.

Coutsoudis, Anna. 2001. "Breast-Feeding and HIV Transmission." *Nutrition Research Reviews* 14, no. 2: 191–206.

Crane, Johanna T., A. Kawuma, Jessica H. Oyugi, J. T. Byakika, Andrew Moss, P. Bourgois, and David R. Bangsberg. 2006. "The Price of Adherence: Qualitative Findings From HIV Positive Individuals Purchasing Fixed-Dose Combination Generic HIV Antiretroviral Therapy in Kampala, Uganda." *AIDS and Behavior* 10, no. 4: 437–442.

Crumbley, Joseph, and Robert Little. 1997. *Relatives Raising Children: An Overview of Kinship Care.* Washington, D.C.: CWLA Press.

Crush, Jonathan, Belinda Dodson, John Gay, Thuso Green, and Clement Leduka. 2010. *Migration, Remittances and "Development" in Lesotho.* Southern African Migration Program, Migration Policy Series 52. Cape Town: Idasa.

Dahl, Bianca. 2014. "'Too Fat to Be an Orphan': The Moral Semiotics of Food Aid in Botswana." *Cultural Anthropology* 29, no. 4: 626–647.

de Walque, Damien, and Rachel Kline. 2012. "The Association between Remarriage and HIV Infection in 13 Sub-Saharan African Countries." *Studies in Family Planning* 43, no. 1: 1–10.

Dilger, Hansjörg, Marian Burchardt, and Rijk van Dijk. 2014. "Religion and AIDS Treatment in Africa: The Redemptive Moment." In *Religion and AIDS Treatment in Africa: Saving Souls, Prolonging Lives,* edited by Rijk van Dijk, Hansjorg Dilger, Marian Burchardt, and Thera Rasing, 1–24. Surrey: Ashgate.

Doherty, Tanya. 2010. "Infant Feeding in the Era of HIV: Challenges and Opportunities." In *Infant Feeding Practices*, edited by Pranee Liamputtong, 175–193. New York: Springer.

Durham, Deborah, and Frederick Klaits. 2002. "Funerals and the Public Space of Sentiment in Botswana." *Journal of Southern African Studies* 28, no. 4: 777–795.

Edkins, Don, Ute Holl, and Michael Schlömer. 1990. *Goldwidows: Women in Lesotho.* DVD. Brooklyn, N.Y.: Icarus Films.

Epprecht, M. 1993. "Domesticity and Piety in Colonial Lesotho: The Private Politics of Basotho Women's Pious Associations." *Journal of Southern African Studies* 19, no. 2: 202–224.

Epstein, Helen. 2007. *The Invisible Cure: Africa, the West, and the Fight against AIDS.* New York: Farrar, Straus and Giroux.

Esu-Williams, E., K. D. Schenk, S. Geibel, J. Motsepe, A. Zulu, P. Bweupe, and E. Weiss. 2006. "'We Are No Longer Called Club Members but Caregivers': Involving Youth in HIV and AIDS Caregiving in Rural Zambia." *AIDS Care* 18, no. 8: 888–894.

Evans-Pritchard, E. E. 1940. *The Nuer: A Description of the Modes of Livelihood and Political Institutions of a Nilotic People.* London: Clarendon Press.

Farmer, Paul. 2001. *Infections and Inequalities: The Modern Plagues.* Berkeley: University of California Press.

———. 2003. "AIDS: A Biosocial Problem with Social Solutions." *Anthropology News* 44, no. 6: 7–7.

———. 2004. "An Anthropology of Structural Violence." *Current Anthropology* 45, no. 3: 305–317.

———. 2009. "On Suffering and Structural Violence: A View from Below." *Race/Ethnicity: Multidisciplinary Global Contexts* 3, no. 1: 11–28.

Fassin, Didier. 2007. *When Bodies Remember: Experiences and Politics of AIDS in South Africa.* Berkeley: University of California Press.

Feeley-Harnik, G. 1980. "The Sakalava House (Madagascar)." *Anthropos* 75, no. 3–4: 559–585.

Ferguson, James. 2006. *Global Shadows: Africa in the Neoliberal World Order.* Durham, N.C.: Duke University Press.

Fisher, William F. 1997. "Doing Good? The Politics and Antipolitics of NGO Practices." *Annual Review of Anthropology* 26, no. 1: 439–464.

Fonseca, Claudia. 2004. "The Circulation of Children in a Brazilian Working-Class Neighborhood." In *Cross-Cultural Approaches to Adoption*, edited by Fiona Bowie, 165–181. New York: Routledge.

Furin, Jennifer. 2011. "The Role of Traditional Healers in Community-Based HIV Care in Rural Lesotho." *Journal of Community Health* 36, no. 5: 849–856.

Geertz, Clifford. 1973. *The Interpretation of Cultures: Selected Essays.* New York: Basic.

Gergen, Kenneth J. 1991. *The Saturated Self: Dilemmas of Identity in Contemporary Life.* New York: Basic.

Gill, Debby. 1994. *The Situation of Children and Women in Lesotho.* Lesotho: Ministry of Planning, Economic, and Manpower Development and UNICEF.

Glick, Peter, and David E. Sahn. 2007. "Changes in HIV/AIDS Knowledge and Testing Behavior in Africa: How Much and for Whom?" *Journal of Population Economics* 20, no. 2: 383–422.

Goodman, Alan H., and Thomas L. Leatherman, eds. 1998. "Traversing the Chasm between Biology and Culture: An Introduction." In *Building a New Biocultural Synthesis: Political-Economic Perspectives on Human Biology*, 3–41. Ann Arbor: University of Michigan Press.

Goody, Esther. 1982. *Parenthood and Social Reproduction: Fostering and Occupational Roles in West Africa.* Cambridge: Cambridge University Press.

————. 1984. "Parental Strategies: Calculation or Sentiment? Fostering Practices among West Africans." In *Interest and Emotion: Essays on the Study of Family and Kinship*, edited by Hans Medick and David Warren Sabean, 266–277. Cambridge: Cambridge University Press.

Gordon, Elizabeth Boltson. 1994. "The Plight of the Women of Lesotho: Reconsideration with the Decline of Apartheid?" *Journal of Black Studies* 24, no. 4: 435–446.

Gottlieb, Geoffrey S., David C. Nickle, Mark A. Jensen, Kim G. Wong, Jandre Grobler, Fusheng Li, Shan-Lu Liu, Cecilia Rademeyer, Gerald H. Learn, Salim S. Abdool Karim, Carolyn Williamson, Lawrence Corey, Joseph B. Margolick, and James I. Mullins. 2004. "Dual HIV-1 Infection Associated with Rapid Disease Progression." *Lancet* 363, no. 9409: 619–622.

Government of Lesotho. 2000. "National AIDS Strategic Plan 2000/2001–2003/2004: A Three-Year Rolling Plan for the National Response to the HIV/AIDS Epidemic in Lesotho." Accessed August 2, 2017. http://www.ilo.org/wcmsp5/groups/public/---ed _protect/---protrav/---ilo_aids/documents/legaldocument/wcms_126750.pdf.

————. 2004. "Guidelines to Prevent Mother-to-Child Transmission of HIV." Accessed June 21, 2018. http://www.ilo.org/wcmsp5/groups/public/---ed_protect/---protrav/ ---ilo_aids/documents/legaldocument/wcms_126758.pdf.

————. 2006. "National HIV and AIDS Strategic Plan (2006–2011)." Accessed June 24, 2018. http://www.aidstar-one.com/sites/default/files/prevention/resources/national _strategic_plans/Lesotho_06-11.pdf.

Grainger, Corinne, Douglas Webb, and Lyn Elliott. 2001. "Children Affected by HIV/AIDS: Rights and Responses in the Developing World." Working Paper 23. London: Save the Children.

Grant, Roy. 2000. "The Special Needs of Children in Kinship Care." *Journal of Gerontological Social Work* 33, no. 3: 17–33.

Green, Edward C. 2003. *Rethinking AIDS Prevention: Learning from Successes in Developing Countries*. Santa Barbara, Calif.: Greenwood.

Green, Edward C., Daniel T. Halperin, Vinand Nantulya, and Janice A. Hogle. 2006. "Uganda's HIV Prevention Success: The Role of Sexual Behavior Change and the National Response." *AIDS and Behavior* 10, no. 4: 335–346.

Grosh, Margaret E., and Paul Glewwe. 1995. *A Guide to Living Standards Measurement Study Surveys and Their Data Sets*. Vol. 120. Washington, D.C.: World Bank.

Guma, Mthobeli. 2001. "The Cultural Meaning of Names among Basotho of Southern Africa: A Historical and Linguistic Analysis." *Nordic Journal of African Studies* 10, no. 3: 265–279.

Gumede-Moyo, Sehlulekile, Suzanne Filteau, Tendai Munthali, Jim Todd, and Patrick Musonda. 2017. "Implementation Effectiveness of Revised (Post-2010) World Health Organization Guidelines on Prevention of Mother-to-Child Transmission of HIV Using Routinely Collected Data in Sub-Saharan Africa: A Systematic Literature Review." *Medicine* 96, no. 40: 1–12.

Hardon, Anita P., Dorothy Akurut, Christopher Comoro, Cosmas Ekezie, Henry F. Irunde, Trudie Gerrits, Joyce Kglatwane et al. 2007. "Hunger, Waiting Time and Transport Costs: Time to Confront Challenges to ART Adherence in Africa." *AIDS Care* 19, no. 5: 658–665.

Hartwig, Kari A., Seelah Kissioki, and Charlotte D. Hartwig. 2006. "Church Leaders Confront HIV/AIDS and Stigma: A Case Study from Tanzania." *Journal of Community & Applied Social Psychology* 16, no. 6: 492–497.

Heidegger, Martin. 1971. "Building Dwelling Thinking." In *Poetry, Language, Thought*, 141–161. New York: Harper & Row.

Henderson, Patricia C. 2011. *AIDS, Intimacy and Care in Rural Kwazulu-Natal: A Kinship of Bones*. Amsterdam: Amsterdam University Press.

Heymann, Jody, Alison Earle, Divya Rajaraman, C. Miller, and Kenneth Bogen. 2007. "Extended Family Caring for Children Orphaned by AIDS: Balancing Essential Work and Caregiving in a High HIV-Prevalence Nations." *AIDS Care* 19, no. 3: 337–345.

Heymann, Jody, and Rachel Kidman. 2009. "HIV/AIDS, Declining Family Resources and the Community Safety Net." *AIDS Care* 21, no. S1: 34–42.

Himmelgreen, David A., Nancy Romero-Daza, David Turkon, Sharon Watson, Ipolto Okello-Uma, and Daniel Sellen. 2009. "Addressing the HIV/AIDS–Food Insecurity Syndemic in Sub-Saharan Africa." *African Journal of AIDS Research* 8, no. 4: 401–412.

Holzemer, William L., Leana Uys, Lucy Makoae, Anita Stewart, René Phetlhu, Priscilla S. Dlamini, Minrie Greeff, Thecla W. Kohi, Maureen Chirwa, and Yvette Cuca. 2007. "A Conceptual Model of HIV/AIDS Stigma from Five African Countries." *Journal of Advanced Nursing* 58, no. 6: 541–551.

Holý, Ladislav. 1996. *Anthropological Perspectives on Kinship*. London: Pluto Press.

HRSA. 2014. "Guide for HIV/AIDS Clinical Care." Accessed June 21, 2018. https://hab.hrsa .gov/sites/default/files/hab/clinical-quality-management/2014guide.pdf.

Hunter, Mark. 2002. "The Materiality of Everyday Sex: Thinking beyond 'Prostitution.'" *African Studies* 61, no. 1: 99–120.

Hutchinson, Sharon. 2000. "Identity and Substance: The Broadening Base of Relatedness among the Nuer of Southern Sudan." In *Cultures of Relatedness: New Approaches to the Study of Kinship*, edited by Janet Carsten, 55–72. Cambridge: Cambridge University Press.

Ingold, Tim. 2000. *The Perception of the Environment: Essays on Livelihood, Dwelling and Skill*. London: Routledge.

Isiugo-Abanihe, U. C. 1985. "Child Fosterage in West Africa." *Population and Development Review* 11, no. 1: 53–73.

Jackson, Cecile. 2015. "Modernity and Matrifocality: The Feminization of Kinship?" *Development and Change* 46, no. 1: 1–24.

Janzen, John M. 1981. "The Need for a Taxonomy of Health in the Study of African Therapeutics." *Social Science and Medicine* 15B, no. 3: 185–194.

———. 1992. *Ngoma: Discourses of Healing in Central and Southern Africa*. Berkeley: University of California Press.

Juma, Laurence. 2011. "The Laws of Lerotholi: Role and Status of Codified Rules of Custom in the Kingdom of Lesotho." *Pace International Law Review* 23, no. 1: 92–145.

Kalichman, Seth C., and Leickness C. Simbayi. 2003. "HIV Testing Attitudes, AIDS Stigma, and Voluntary HIV Counselling and Testing in a Black Township in Cape Town, South Africa." *Sexually Transmitted Infections* 79, no. 6: 442–447.

———. 2004. "Traditional Beliefs about the Cause of AIDS and AIDS-Related Stigma in South Africa." *AIDS Care* 16, no. 5: 572–580.

Karp, Ivan. 1980. "Beer Drinking and Social Experience in an African Society: An Essay in Formal Sociology." In *Explorations in African Systems of Thought*, edited by Ivan Karp and Charles S. Bird, 83–119. Bloomington: Indiana University Press.

Kaufman, Carol E. 2004. "'Bus Fare Please': The Economics of Sex and Gifts among Young People in Urban South Africa." *Culture, Health and Sexuality* 6, no. 5: 377–391.

Kelly, Jeffrey A., Anton M. Somlai, Eric G. Benotsch, Yuri A. Amirkhanian, Maria I. Fernandez, L. Y. Stevenson, Cheryl A. Sitzler, Timothy L. Mcauliffe, Kevin D. Brown, and Karen M. Opgenorth. 2006. "Programmes, Resources, and Needs of HIV-Prevention

Nongovernmental Organizations (NGOs) in Africa, Central/Eastern Europe and Central Asia, Latin America and the Caribbean." *AIDS Care* 18, no. 1: 12–21.

Kenworthy, Nora J. 2017. *Mistreated: The Political Consequences of the Fight against AIDS in Lesotho.* Nashville, Tenn.: Vanderbilt University Press.

Kenworthy, Nora, Matthew Thomann, and Richard Parker. 2017. "From a Global Crisis to the 'End of AIDS': New Epidemics of Signification." *Global Public Health* 13, no. 8: 1–12.

Kimble, Judy. 1982. "Labour Migration in Basutoland, c. 1870–1885." In *Industrialisation and Social Change in South Africa: African Class Formation, Culture, and Consciousness, 1870–1930,* edited by Shula Marks and Richard Rathbone, 119–141. London: Longman.

Kimemia, V. Muthoni. 2006. "Caregiver Burden and Coping Responses for Females Who Are the Primary Caregiver for a Family Member Living with HIV/AIDS in Kenya." PhD diss., University of South Florida.

Kipp, Walter, Thomas Matukala Nkosi, Lory Laing, and Gian Jhangri. 2006. "Care Burden and Self-Reported Health Status of Informal Women Caregivers of HIV/AIDS Patients in Kinshasa, Democratic Republic of Congo." *AIDS Care* 18, no. 7: 694–697.

Klaits, Frederick. 2010. *Death in a Church Life: Moral Passion during Botswana's Time of AIDS.* Berkeley: University of California Press.

Kleinman, Arthur. 1980. *Patients and Healers in the Context of Culture: An Exploration of the Borderland between Anthropology, Medicine, and Psychiatry.* Berkeley: University of California Press.

———. 2009. "Caregiving: The Odyssey of Becoming More Human." *Lancet* 373, no. 9660: 292–293.

———. 2012. "Caregiving as Moral Experience." *Lancet* 380, no. 985: 1550–1551.

Kwansa, Benjamin Kobina. 2014. "'Silent Nights, Anointing Days': Post-HIV Test Religious Experiences in Ghana." In *Religion and AIDS Treatment in Africa: Saving Souls, Prolonging Lives,* edited by Rijk van Dijk, Hansjorg Dilger, Marian Burchardt, and Thera Rasing, 147–168. Surrey: Ashgate.

Langwick, Stacey Ann. 2011. *Bodies, Politics, and African Healing: The Matter of Maladies in Tanzania.* Bloomington: Indiana University Press.

Larsson, Anita. 1996. "Housing Conflicts and Women's Strategies in Lesotho." In *A Place to Live: Gender Research on Housing in Africa,* edited by Ann Schlyter, 64–76. Uppsala: Nordic Africa Institute.

Leatherman, Tom, and Alan H. Goodman. 2011. "Critical Biocultural Approaches in Medical Anthropology." In *A Companion to Medical Anthropology,* edited by Merrill Singer and Pamela I. Erickson, 29–48. West Sussex: John Wiley and Sons.

Leclerc-Madlala, S. 2003. "Transactional Sex and the Pursuit of Modernity." *Social Dynamics* 9, no. 2: 213–233.

Leduka, Resetselemang, Jonathan Crush, Bruce Frayne, Cameron McCordic, Thope Matobo, Ts'episo E. Makoa, Matseliso Mphale, Mmantai Phaila, and Moipone Letsie. 2015. *The State of Poverty and Food Insecurity in Maseru, Lesotho.* AFSUN Urban Food Security Series 21. Cape Town: African Food Security Urban Network.

Leinaweaver, Jessaca. 2005. "Familiar Ways: Child Circulation in Andean Peru." PhD diss., University of Michigan.

———. 2007. "On Moving Children: The Social Implications of Andean Child Circulation." *American Ethnologist* 34, no. 1: 163–180.

———. 2008. *The Circulation of Children: Kinship, Adoption, and Morality in Andean Peru.* Durham, N.C.: Duke University Press.

————. 2014. "Informal Kinship-Based Fostering around the World: Anthropological Findings." *Child Development Perspectives* 8, no. 3: 131–136.

Lesotho Bureau of Statistics. 2008. "Lesotho Integrated Labour Force Survey." Accessed May 24, 2018. http://catalog.ihsn.org/index.php/catalog/4531/download/57895.

————. 2016. "Lesotho Census Summary Key Findings." Accessed May 24, 2018. http://www.bos.gov.ls/2016%20Summary%20Key%20Findings.pdf.

Lesotho Ministry of Health. 2005. "Lesotho Demographic and Health Survey 2004: Preliminary Report." Accessed April 22, 2018. https://www.dhsprogram.com/pubs/pdf/FR171/FR171.pdf.

————. 2010. "Lesotho Demographic and Health Survey 2009." Accessed May 21, 2018. http://pdf.usaid.gov/pdf_docs/PNADU407.pdf.

————. 2011. "Distribution of Hospitals and Clinics in Lesotho." Accessed July 12, 2017. http://www.health.gov.ls/index.php?option=com_content&view=article&id=31:facil.

————. 2015. "Global AIDS Response Progress Report 2015: Follow-Up to the 2011 Political Declaration on HIV/AIDS Intensifying Efforts to Eliminate HIV/AIDS." Accessed May 24, 2018. http://www.unaids.org/sites/default/files/country/documents/LSO_narrative_report_2015.pdf.

————. 2016. "Lesotho Demographic and Health Survey 2014." Accessed June 21, 2018. https://www.dhsprogram.com/pubs/pdf/FR309/FR309.pdf.

Lesotho Ministry of Local Government and Chieftainship. 2012. "Mission/Vision/Values." Accessed August 13, 2017. http://www.gov.ls/ministry-of-local-government-and-chieftainship/.

Liddell, Christine, Louise Barrett, and Moya Bydawell. 2005. "Indigenous Representations of Illness and AIDS in Sub-Saharan Africa." *Social Science and Medicine* 60, no. 4: 691–700.

Lincoln, Yvonna S., and Egon G. Guba. 1985. *Naturalistic Inquiry.* Beverly Hills, Calif.: Sage.

Livingston, Julie. 2012. *Improvising Medicine: An African Oncology Ward in an Emerging Cancer Epidemic.* Durham, N.C.: Duke University Press.

Lock, Margaret. 1993. "Cultivating the Body: Anthropology and Epistemologies of Bodily Practice and Knowledge." *Annual Review of Anthropology* 22, no. 1: 133–155.

————. 2001. "The Tempering of Medical Anthropology: Troubling Natural Categories." *Medical Anthropology Quarterly* 15, no. 4: 478–492.

Lock, Margaret M., and Patricia A. Kaufert, eds. 1998. Introduction to *Pragmatic Women and Body Politics,* 1–27. Cambridge: Cambridge University Press.

Lévi-Strauss, Claude. 1969. *The Elementary Structures of Kinship.* Boston: Beacon Press.

Mah, Timothy L., and Daniel T. Halperin. 2010. "Concurrent Sexual Partnerships and the HIV Epidemics in Africa: Evidence to Move Forward." *AIDS and Behavior* 14, no. 1: 11–16.

Mahajan, Anish P., Jennifer N. Sayles, Vishal A. Patel, Robert H. Remien, Daniel Ortiz, Greg Szekeres, and Thomas J. Coates. 2008. "Stigma in the HIV/AIDS Epidemic: A Review of the Literature and Recommendations for the Way Forward." *AIDS* 22, no. S2: S67–S79.

Manderson, Lenore, and Ellen Block. 2016. "Relatedness and Care in Southern Africa and Beyond." *Social Dynamics* 42, no. 2: 205–217.

Manderson, Lenore, Ellen Block, and Nolwazi Mkhwanazi. 2016. "Fragility, Fluidity, and Resilience: Caregiving Configurations Three Decades into AIDS." *AIDS Care* 28, no. S4: 1–7.

Mapetla, Matseliso M. 2009. *SADC Gender Protocol Barometer Baseline Study: Lesotho.* Roma: National University of Lesotho.

Mayosi, Bongani M., and Solomon R. Benatar. 2014. "Health and Health Care in South Africa—20 Years after Mandela." *New England Journal of Medicine* 371, no. 14: 1344–1353.

McAllister, Patrick A. 1993. "Indigenous Beer in Southern Africa—Functions and Fluctuations." *African Studies* 52, no. 1: 71–88.

McMichael, Anthony J. 1995. "The Health of Persons, Populations, and Planets: Epidemiology Comes Full Circle." *Epidemiology* 6, no. 6: 633–636.

Médecins Sans Frontières. 2007. "Help Wanted: Confronting the Healthcare Worker Crisis to Expand Access to HIV/AIDS Treatment." Accessed August 8, 2017. https://www.msf.org/help-wanted-confronting-health-care-worker-crisis.

Merten, Sonja. 2016. "Ambiguous Care: Siblings and the Economies of HIV-Related Care in Zambia." *AIDS Care* 28, no. S4: 41–50.

Mfecane, Sakhumzi. 2012. "Narratives of HIV Disclosure and Masculinity in a South African Village." *Culture, Health and Sexuality* 14, no. S1: S109–S121.

Miller, Daniel. 2001. *Home Possessions: Material Culture behind Closed Doors.* Oxford: Berg.

Mills, Edward J., Jean B. Nachega, Iain Buchan, James Orbinski, Amir Attaran, Sonal Singh, Beth Rachlis, Ping Wu, Curtis Cooper, Lehana Thabane, Kumanan Wilson, Gordon H. Guyatt, and D. R. Bangsberg. 2006. "Adherence to Antiretroviral Therapy in Sub-Saharan Africa and North America: A Meta-analysis." *JAMA* 296, no. 6: 679–690.

Modo, I. V. O. 2001. "The Changing Family Structure and Legal Lag in Lesotho: Implications for the Future." *African Anthropologist* 8, no. 1: 69–84.

Mol, Annemarie. 2008. *The Logic of Care: Health and the Problem of Patient Choice.* London: Routledge.

Mol, Annemarie, Ingunn Moser, and Jeannette Pols. 2010. "Care: Putting Practice into Theory." In *Care in Practice: On Tinkering in Clinics, Homes and Farms*, edited by Annemarie Mol, Ingunn Moser, and Jeannette Pols, 7–26. Bielefeld: Transcript Verlag.

Morton, Christopher. 2007. "Remembering the House: Memory and Materiality in Northern Botswana." *Journal of Material Culture* 12, no. 2: 157–179.

Moscovici, Serge. 2001. *Social Representations: Essays in Social Psychology.* New York: NYU Press.

Moshabela, M., P. Pronyk, N. Williams, H. Schneider, and M. Lurie. 2011. "Patterns and Implications of Medical Pluralism among HIV/AIDS Patients in Rural South Africa." *AIDS and Behavior* 15, no. 4: 842–852.

Murray, Colin. 1976. "Marital Strategy in Lesotho: The Redistribution of Migrant Earnings." *African Studies* 35, no. 2: 99–122.

———. 1981. *Families Divided: The Impact of Migrant Labour in Lesotho.* Cambridge: Cambridge University Press.

Mwase, Takondwa, Eddie Kariisa, Julie Doherty, Nomaphuthi Hoohlo-Khotle, Paul Kiwanuka-Mukiibi, and Taylor Williamson. 2010. "Lesotho Health Systems Assessment." Bethesda, Md.: Health Systems 20/20.

Nachega, Jean B., D. M. Stein, D. A. Lehman, D. Hlatshwayo, R. Mothopeng, R. E. Chaisson, and A. S. Karstaedt. 2004. "Adherence to Antiretroviral Therapy in HIV-Infected Adults in Soweto, South Africa." *AIDS Research and Human Retroviruses* 20, no. 10: 1053–1056.

Ncama, Busisiwe P., Patricia A. McInerney, Busisiwe R. Bhengu, Inge B. Corless, Dean J. Wantland, Patrice K. Nicholas, Chris A. McGibbon, and Sheila M. Davis. 2008. "Social Support and Medication Adherence in HIV Disease in KwaZulu-Natal, South Africa." *International Journal of Nursing Studies* 45, no. 12: 1757–1763.

Negin, Joel, and Robert G. Cumming. 2010. "HIV Infection in Older Adults in Sub-Saharan Africa: Extrapolating Prevalence from Existing Data." *Bulletin of the World Health Organization* 88, no. 11: 847–853.

Negin, Joel, Edward J. Mills, and Rachel Albone. 2011. "Continued Neglect of Ageing of HIV Epidemic at UN Meeting." *Lancet* 378, no. 9793: 768.

Nguyen, Vinh-Kim. 2005. "Antiretroviral Globalism, Biopolitics, and Therapeutic Citizenship." In *Global Assemblages: Technology, Politics, and Ethics as Anthropological Problems*, edited by Stephen J. Collier and Aihwa Ong, 124–144. Oxford: Blackwell.

Nora, Pierre. 1989. "Between Memory and History: Les Lieux de Mémoire." *Representations* 26:7–24.

Ntimo-Makara, Matora. 2009. *Living with Divorce: Expectations and Contradictions within the Lesotho Socio-cultural Context*. Addis Ababa: OSSREA.

Nxumalo, Nonhlanhla, Jane Goudge, and Lenore Manderson. 2016. "Community Health Workers, Recipients' Experiences and Constraints to Care in South Africa: A Pathway to Trust." *AIDS Care* 28, no. S4: 61–71.

Nyambedha, Erick O., Simiyu Wandibba, and Jens Aagaard-Hansen. 2003. "Retirement Lost: The New Role of the Elderly as Caretakers for Orphans in Western Kenya." *Journal of Cross-Cultural Gerontology* 18, no. 1: 33–52.

Obasi, A. I., B. Cleophas, D. A. Ross, K. L. Chima, G. Mmassy, A. Gavyole, M. L. Plummer, M. Makokha, M. Mujaya, J. Todd, D. Wight, H. Grosskurth, D. C. Mabey, and R. J. Hayes. 2006. "Rationale and Design of the MEMA kwa Vijana Adolescent Sexual and Reproductive Health Intervention in Mwanza Region, Tanzania." *AIDS Care* 18, no. 4: 311–322.

Obioha, Emeka E., and Nete Khoanyane. 2012. "An Anthropological Investigation of Sotho Worldviews, Myths and Stereotypes Attached to Immigrants in Lesotho, Southern Africa." *Anthropologist* 14, no. 5: 473–483.

Oladokun, Regina E., Biobele J. Brown, and Kikelomo Osinusi. 2010. "Infant-Feeding Pattern of HIV-Positive Women in a Prevention of Mother-to-Child Transmission (PMTCT) Programme." *AIDS Care* 22, no. 9: 1108–1114.

Olsen, Bjørnar. 2010. *In Defense of Things: Archaeology and the Ontology of Objects*. Lanham, Md.: AltaMira Press.

Ortner, Sherry B. 1984. "Theory in Anthropology since the Sixties." *Comparative Studies in Society and History* 26, no. 1: 126–166.

Owusu-Ampomah, Kwame, Scott Naysmith, and Cara Rubincam. 2009. "Reviewing 'Emergencies' in HIV and AIDS-Affected Countries in Southern Africa: Shifting the Paradigm in Lesotho." Accessed February 3, 2018. https://www.k4health.org/sites/default/files/lesotho_emergencies_report_final.pdf.

Page, Hilary. 1989. "Childrearing versus Childbearing: Coresidence of Mother and Child in Sub-Saharan Africa." In *Reproduction and Social Organization in Sub-Saharan Africa*, edited by Ron J. Lesthaeghe, 401–441. Berkeley: University of California Press.

Parikh, Shanti A. 2007. "The Political Economy of Marriage and HIV: The ABC Approach, 'Safe' Infidelity, and Managing Moral Risk in Uganda." *American Journal of Public Health* 97, no. 7: 1198–1208.

Parker, Richard. 2001. "Sexuality, Culture, and Power in HIV/AIDS Research." *Annual Review of Anthropology* 30, no. 1: 163–179.

Parsitau, Damaris Seleina. 2009. "'Keep Holy Distance and Abstain till He Comes': Interrogating a Pentecostal Church's Engagements with HIV/AIDS and the Youth in Kenya." *Africa Today* 56, no. 1: 45–64.

Pearce, Tola. 1995. "Women's Reproductive Practices and Biomedicine: Cultural Conflicts and Transformations in Nigeria." In *Conceiving the New World Order: The Global Politics of Reproduction*, edited by F. D. Ginsburg and Rayna Rapp, 195–208. Berkeley: University of California Press.

Peletz, Michael G. 1995. "Kinship Studies in Late Twentieth-Century Anthropology." *Annual Review of Anthropology* 24, no. 1: 343–372.

Peltzer, Karl, Natalie Friend-du Preez, Shandir Ramlagan, Henry Fomundam, and Jane Anderson. 2010. "Traditional Complementary and Alternative Medicine and Antiretroviral Treatment Adherence among HIV Patients in KwaZulu-Natal, South Africa." *African Journal of Traditional, Complementary, and Alternative Medicines* 7, no. 2: 125–137.

Peltzer, Karl, Natalie Friend-du Preez, Shandir Ramlagan, and Henry Fomundam. 2008. "Use of Traditional Complementary and Alternative Medicine for HIV Patients in KwaZulu-Natal, South Africa." *BMC Public Health* 8, no. 1: 255–268.

Peluso, Nancy Lee. 1996. "Fruit Trees and Family Trees in an Anthropogenic Forest: Ethics of Access, Property Zones, and Environmental Change in Indonesia." *Comparative Studies in Society and History* 38, no. 3: 510–548.

Pfeiffer, J., and M. Nichter. 2008. "What Can Critical Medical Anthropology Contribute to Global Health?" *Medical Anthropology Quarterly* 22, no. 4: 410–415.

Prazak, Miroslava. 2012. "Studying Life Strategies of AIDS Orphans in Rural Kenya." *Africa Today* 58, no. 4: 44–64.

Prince, Ruth. 2009. "Introduction to Special Issue: Engaging Christianities: Negotiating HIV/AIDS, Health, and Social Relations in East and Southern Africa." *Africa Today* 56, no. 1: v–xviii.

Radcliffe-Brown, A. R., and Cyril Daryll Forde, eds. 1951. *African Systems of Kinship and Marriage*. London: Oxford University Press.

Ramashwar, S. 2012. "Remarriage, HIV Infection Linked among Women in Sub-Saharan Africa." *International Perspectives on Sexual and Reproductive Health* 38, no. 2: 113–114.

Ramphele, Mamphela. 1993. *A Bed Called Home: Life in the Migrant Labour Hostels of Cape Town*. Athens: Ohio University Press.

Renne, Elisha P. 1993. "History in the Making: An Anthropological Approach to the Demographic Analysis of Child Fostering in Southwestern Nigeria." *IUSSP General Population Conference* 3:327–342.

———. 2003. *Population and Progress in a Yoruba Town*. Ann Arbor: University of Michigan Press.

Robbins, Joel. 2013. "Beyond the Suffering Subject: Toward an Anthropology of the Good." *Journal of the Royal Anthropological Institute* 19, no. 3: 447–462.

Robins, Steven. 2008. "Sexual Politics and the Zuma Rape Trial." *Journal of Southern African Studies* 34, no. 2: 411–427.

Robson, Elsbeth, Nicola Ansell, U. S. Huber, W. T. S. Gould, and Lorraine van Blerk. 2006. "Young Caregivers in the Context of the HIV/AIDS Pandemic in Sub-Saharan Africa." *Population, Space and Place* 12, no. 2: 93–111.

Romero-Daza, Nancy. 2002. "Traditional Medicine in Africa." *Annals of the American Academy of Political and Social Science* 583, no. 1: 173–176.

Romero-Daza, Nancy, and David Himmelgreen. 1998. "More Than Money for Your Labor: Migration and the Political Economy of AIDS in Lesotho." In *The Political Economy of AIDS*, edited by Merrill Singer, 185–204. Amityville, N.Y.: Baywood.

Saul, M. 1981. "Beer, Sorghum and Women: Production for the Market in Rural Upper Volta." *Africa* 51, no. 3: 746–764.

Sakarovitch, Charlotte, Francois Rouet, Gary Murphy, Albert K. Minga, Ahmadou Alioum, Francois Dabis, Dominique Costagliola, Roger Salamon, John V. Parry, and Francis Barin. 2007. "Do Tests Devised to Detect Recent HIV-1 Infection Provide Reliable Estimates of Incidence in Africa?" *JAIDS* 45, no. 1: 115–122.

Samji, Hasina, Angela Cescon, Robert S. Hogg, Sharada P. Modur, Keri N. Althoff, Kate Buchacz, Ann N. Burchell, Mardge Cohen, Kelly A. Gebo, and M. John Gill. 2013. "Closing the Gap: Increases in Life Expectancy among Treated HIV-Positive Individuals in the United States and Canada." *PLOS ONE* 8, no. 12: e81355.

Schiltz, Marie-Ange, and Theodorus G. M. Sandfort. 2000. "HIV-Positive People, Risk and Sexual Behaviour." *Social Science and Medicine* 50, no. 11: 1571–1588.

Schrauwers, A. 1999. "Negotiating Parentage: The Political Economy of 'Kinship' in Central Sulawesi, Indonesia." *American Ethnologist* 26, no. 2: 310–323.

Schwitters, Amee M. 2017. "Notes from the Field: Preliminary Results after Implementation of a Universal Treatment Program (Test and Start) for Persons Living with HIV Infection—Lesotho—October 2015–February 2017." *Morbidity and Mortality Weekly Report* 66, no. 30: 813–814.

Sekatle, Pontso Matumelo. 2011. "Legal Notice No. 21 of 2011: Land Regulations, 2011." Accessed March 9, 2012. http://www.laa.org.ls/download/land-regulations-2011/#.

Shiffman, Jeremy. 2009. "A Social Explanation for the Rise and Fall of Global Health Issues." *Bulletin of the World Health Organization* 87, no. 8: 608–613.

Sidley, Pat. 2001. "Drug Companies Sue South African Government over Generics." *British Medical Journal* 322, no. 7284: 447.

Singer, M. 1989. "The Coming of Age of Critical Medical Anthropology." *Social Science and Medicine* 28, no. 11: 1193–1203.

Singh, Dinesh, Stephenie Chaudoir, Maria Cabrera Escobar, and Seth Kalichman. 2011. "Stigma, Burden, Social Support, and Willingness to Care among Caregivers of PLWHA in Home-Based Care in South Africa." *AIDS Care* 23, no. 7: 1–845.

Skinner, Donald, and Sakhumzi Mfecane. 2004. "Stigma, Discrimination and the Implications for People Living with HIV/AIDS in South Africa." *SAHARA* 1, no. 3: 157–164.

Smith, Daniel Jordan. 2014. *AIDS Doesn't Show Its Face: Inequality, Morality, and Social Change in Nigeria.* Chicago: University of Chicago Press.

Spiegel, Andrew D. 1981. "Changing Patterns of Migrant Labour and Rural Differentiation in Lesotho." *Social Dynamics* 6, no. 2: 1–13.

Steer, Philip. 2005. "The Epidemiology of Preterm Labor: A Global Perspective." *Journal of Perinatal Medicine* 33, no. 4: 273–276.

Suzman, Susan M. 1994. "Names as Pointers: Zulu Personal Naming Practices." *Language in Society* 23, no. 2: 253–272.

Tanga, Pius Tangwe. 2013. "The Challenges of Social Work Field Training in Lesotho." *Social Work Education* 32, no. 2: 157–178.

Taylor, Julie J. 2007. "Assisting or Compromising Intervention? The Concept of 'Culture' in Biomedical and Social Research on HIV/AIDS." *Social Science and Medicine* 64, no. 4: 965–975.

Timaeus, Ian, and Wendy Graham. 1989. "Labor Circulation Marriage and Fertility in Southern Africa." In *Reproduction and Social Organization in Sub-Saharan Africa*, edited by Ron J. Lesthaeghe, 365–400. Berkeley: University of California Press.

Townsend, Loraine, and Andy Dawes. 2004. "Willingness to Care for Children Orphaned by HIV/AIDS: A Study of Foster and Adoptive Parents." *African Journal of AIDS Research* 3, no. 1: 69–80.

Townsend, Nicholas W. 1997. "Men, Migration, and Households in Botswana: An Exploration of Connections over Time and Space." *Journal of Southern African Studies* 23, no. 3: 405–420.

Turkon, David. 2003. "Modernity, Tradition and the Demystification of Cattle in Lesotho." *African Studies* 62, no. 2: 147–169.

Turkon, David, David Himmelgreen, Nancy Romero-Daza, and Charlotte Noble. 2009. "Anthropological Perspectives on the Challenges to Monitoring and Evaluating HIV and AIDS Programming in Lesotho." *African Journal of AIDS Research* 8, no. 4: 473–480.

UNAIDS. 2010. "Lesotho UNGASS Country Report: Status of the National Response to the 2001 Declaration of Commitment on HIV and AIDS." Accessed January 26, 2018. http://data.unaids.org/pub/report/2010/lesotho_2010_country_progress_report_en.pdf.

———. 2012. "Lesotho Global AIDS Response Country Progress Report." Accessed June 26, 2018. http://www.unaids.org/sites/default/files/country/documents/file,68395,fr.pdf.

———. 2014. "AIDS Info Data Sheet." Accessed April 17, 2018. http://aidsinfo.unaids.org/.

———. 2016. "Press Release: UNAIDS Warns That after Significant Reductions, Declines in New HIV Infections among Adults Have Stalled and Are Rising in Some Regions." Accessed March 10, 2018. http://www.unaids.org/en/resources/presscentre/pressrelease andstatementarchive/2016/july/20160712_prevention-gap.

———. 2017. "UNAIDS Data 2017." Accessed February 25, 2018. http://www.unaids.org/sites/default/files/media_asset/20170720_Data_book_2017_en.pdf.

UNDP. 2013. "Millennium Development Goals Status Report." Accessed March 30, 2017. http://www.undp.org/content/dam/undp/library/MDG/english/MDG%20Country %20Reports/Lesotho/LESOTHO%20MDGR%202013%20-%20FINAL.pdf.

UNICEF. 2009. "Lesotho: Strengthening Child Protection Services for Survivors of Sexual Abuse." Accessed June 26, 2018. https://www.unicef.org/innovations/index_49367 .html.

Van der Vliet, Virginia, Kyle D. Kauffman, and David L. Lindauer. 2004. *AIDS and South Africa: The Social Expression of a Pandemic*. New York: Palgrave Macmillan.

Wainaina, Binyavanga. 2006. "How to Write about Africa." *Granta* 96. Accessed June 26, 2018. https://granta.com/how-to-write-about-africa/.

Walmsley, Emily. 2008. "Raised by Another Mother: Informal Fostering and Kinship Ambiguities in Northwest Ecuador." *Journal of Latin American and Caribbean Anthropology* 13, no. 1: 168–195.

Weigel, Jonathan, Matthew Basilico, Vanessa Kerry, Madeleine Ballard, Anne Becker, Gene Bukhman, Ophelia Dahl, Andy Ellner, Louise Ivers, David Jones, John Meara, Joia Mukherjee, Amy Sievers, Alyssa Yamamoto, and Paul Farmer. 2013. "Global Health Priorities for the Early Twenty-First Century." In *Reimagining Global Health: An Introduction*, edited by Paul Farmer, Arthur Kleinman, Jim Kim, and Matthew Basilico, 302–339. Berkeley: University of California Press.

Wendland, Claire. 2010. *A Heart for the Work: Journeys through an African Medical School*. Chicago: University of Chicago Press.

Weston, Kath. 1991. *Families We Choose: Lesbians, Gays, Kinship*. New York: Columbia University Press.

WHO. 2005. "Lesotho Summary Country Profile for HIV/AIDS Treatment Scale-Up." Accessed October 18, 2017. http://www.who.int/hiv/HIVCP_LSO.pdf.

———. 2006. "Working Together for Health: The World Health Report 2006." Accessed March 30, 2018. http://www.who.int/whr/2006/en/.

———. 2009. "New HIV Recommendations to Improve Health, Reduce Infection and Save Lives." Accessed June 26, 2018. http://www.who.int/mediacentre/news/releases/2009/world_aids_20091130/en/index.html.

———. 2012. "Mother-to-Child Transmission of HIV." Accessed January 15, 2018. http://www.who.int/hiv/topics/mtct/en/.

———. 2014. "Noncommunicable Diseases Country Profiles: Lesotho." Accessed May 24, 2018. http://www.who.int/nmh/countries/lso_en.pdf.

Yanagisako, Sylvia Junko. 1979. "Family and Household: The Analysis of Domestic Groups." *Annual Review of Anthropology* 8, no. 1: 161–205.

Young, Lorraine, and Nicola Ansell. 2003. "Fluid Households, Complex Families: The Impacts of Children's Migration as a Response to HIV/AIDS in Southern Africa." *Professional Geographer* 55, no. 4: 464–476.

Young, Sera, Amanda C. Wheeler, Sandra I. McCoy, and Sheri D. Weiser. 2014. "A Review of the Role of Food Insecurity in Adherence to Care and Treatment among Adult and Pediatric Populations Living with HIV and AIDS." *AIDS and Behavior* 18, no. 5: 505–515.

Zagheni, E. 2011. "The Impact of the HIV/AIDS Epidemic on Kinship Resources for Orphans in Zimbabwe." *Population and Development Review* 37, no. 4: 761–783.

Zimmerman, Mary K., Jacquelyn S. Litt, and Christine E. Bose. 2006. Introduction to *Global Dimensions of Gender and Carework*, edited by Mary K. Zimmerman, Jacquelyn S. Litt, and Christine E. Bose, 1–6. Stanford, Calif.: Stanford Social Sciences.

# INDEX

abstinence: and churches, 116, 130, 203n3 (chap. 2); and HIV prevention, 128

adherence (HIV): in Africa, 90; barriers to, 92, 102, 139, 146–147, 169; and food insecurity, 56; government sessions, 14, 92, 121–123; monitoring, 15, 31, 85; and treatment failure, 15, 147

Adichie, Chimamanda Ngozi, xvii–xix

adoption, 19, 38, 167, 191–192

affection. *See* love

affinal kin, 56–59; and bridewealth, 74–75, 176; and care, 168–169; and naming practices, 42; and obligations, 20, 132; and patrilineality, 20; and relatedness, 50; tensions between, 48, 173–174; and tension with mothers-in-law, 58–59, 64. *See also* bridewealth

agriculture. *See* farming

AIDS knowledge, 89, 112–128, 134; and biomedicine, 95, 101, 112; and elderly, 124–128; impact on care, 124; and symptom focus, 90–93. *See also* HIV/AIDS

Alber, Erdmute, 161, 172

ancestors: food sharing with, 17, 52, 55; and houses, 41, 72; and kinship, 41; and naming practices, 40, 49

antenatal care, 136, 137

anthropology of the good, xvii, xix, 189

antiretroviral treatment. *See* treatment

ART. *See* treatment

ARVs. *See* treatment

beer. *See joala*

Benton, Adia, 186

biocultural, 15, 94, 144, 145, 190

biomedicine: availability of, 83–86, 93; importance of, 92, 94, 101, 104, 111–113; limits of, 7, 87, 90, 93, 94, 145, 185; preference for, 82, 93–103, 124. *See also* disease etiologies; doctors; nurses

blood: cross-cultural conceptions of, 50–51; and HIV, 122, 123, 150; Sesotho conceptions of, 50; as shared substance, 45

Borneman, John, 158–173

Bourdieu, Pierre, 20, 66, 158, 190. *See also* practice theory

Bray, Rachel, 160

breastfeeding: examples of, 24, 26; and HIV, 56, 121, 136, 138, 139; significance of, 50–52, 138. *See also* milk; substances

breastmilk. *See* breastfeeding; milk

bridewealth (*likhomo*), 17, 62–65; decline in, 58, 62–64, 73, 75, 188; and elderly vs. young people, 176–177; importance of, 62, 157; and marriage, 57–60, 65; and orphan care, 23, 41, 172–176, 178; and patrilineality, 21, 38

Bulled, Nicola, 115

Butler, Judith, 173

care: for AIDS orphans, 16–18, 23, 113, 167–172; "bad" care, 161, 164, 170–172, 177; centrality of, xv, 18, 38, 66, 74, 91, 190; by elderly, 124–128; for elderly, 17; "good," 39–40, 163–165; for HIV-positive adults, 18, 61, 122, 126; for HIV-positive children, 15, 97, 113, 136, 138, 146–147, 167–172; impact of AIDS on, 17, 73, 86–87, 89, 151, 178; intergenerational, 160–164; kin-based, xv, 16–17, 74–75, 91, 158, 192–194; and kinship, 38–40, 74, 158, 189; labor of, 40, 65, 73, 158; and morality, 39, 146, 166, 178; by nonkin, 38, 45, 166, 167; and poverty, 158, 164–165, 167, 172, 178; and practice, 20–22, 39–40. *See also* caregivers; fostering; houses; love; matrilocal care; orphans; patrilineality

caregivers: burden on, 15, 145, 192; changes in, 17, 165–166; elderly, 27, 124–128, 192; grandmothers as, 113, 158, 162–163, 165–167, 191–194; impact of AIDS on, 6,

# ABOUT THE AUTHORS

ELLEN BLOCK is an assistant professor of anthropology in the department of sociology at the College of Saint Benedict and Saint John's University in Collegeville, Minnesota.

WILL MCGRATH is an award-winning writer and journalist. He has written for the *Atlantic, Pacific Standard, Foreign Affairs,* the *Christian Science Monitor,* and *Gastronomica.* He is also the author of *Everything Lost Is Found Again.*